Current Concepts in Arrhythmogenic Right Ventricular Cardiomyopathy/Dysplasia

Current Concepts in Arrhythmogenic Right Ventricular Cardiomyopathy/Dysplasia

Editors:

Prof. Dr. CORINNA BRUNCKHORST, MD
Co-Director Arrhythmia Service
University Heart Center, Zurich, Switzerland

Prof. Dr. FIRAT DURU, MD
Director Arrhythmia Service
University Heart Center, Zurich, Switzerland

Associate Editor:

Dr. ARDAN M. SAGUNER, MD
Fellow Arrhythmia Service
University Heart Center, Zurich, Switzerland

cardiotext®
PUBLISHING
Minneapolis, Minnesota

Cardiotext Publishing, LLC
3405 W. 44th Street
Minneapolis, Minnesota 55410
USA

www.cardiotextpublishing.com

Any updates to this book may be found at: www.cardiotextpublishing.com/arvc-d/

Comments, inquiries, and requests for bulk sales can be directed to the publisher at: info@cardiotextpublishing.com.

Library of Congress Control Number: 2014933127

ISBN: 978-1-935395-92-8

eISBN: 978-1-935395-19-5

Printed in the United States of America

Dedication

We thank our families for their support and understanding.

We dedicate this book to all patients with arrhythmogenic right ventricular cardiomyopathy/dysplasia. We hope that it serves as a source of knowledge and inspiration for the physicians and scientists who aim to provide the best medical care for patients with this disease. We are grateful to the Georg and Bertha Schwyzer-Winiker Foundation for supporting the Zurich ARVC Program and for making this book possible.

—The Editors

Table of Contents

Contributors

Editors

Prof. Dr. Corinna Brunckhorst, MD
Co-Director Arrhythmia Service, University Heart Center, Zurich, Switzerland

Prof. Dr. Firat Duru, MD
Director Arrhythmia Service, University Heart Center, Zurich, Switzerland

Associate Editor

Ardan M. Saguner, MD
Fellow Arrhythmia Service, University Heart Center, Zurich, Switzerland

Contributors

Esperanza Agullo-Pascual, PhD
Leon H. Charney Division of Cardiology, New York University School of Medicine, New York, New York, USA

Hugh Calkins, MD
Professor of Medicine, Nicholas J. Fortuin Professor of Cardiology, Johns Hopkins Medical Institutions, Johns Hopkins, Baltimore, Maryland, USA

Marina Cerrone, MD
Cardiovascular Genetics Program, Leon H. Charney Division of Cardiology, New York University School of Medicine, New York, New York, USA

Domenico Corrado, MD, PhD
Division of Cardiology, Inherited Arrhythmogenic Cardiomyopathy Unit, Department of Cardiac, Thoracic and Vascular Sciences, University of Padua, Italy

Mario Delmar, MD, PhD
Professor of Medicine/Cardiology, Leon H. Charney Division of Cardiology, New York University School of Medicine, New York, New York, USA

Paul Erne, MD
CardioVasc Schweiz, Klinik St. Anna, Lucerne, Switzerland; Department of Cardiology, University Heart Center, Zurich, Switzerland

Guy H. Fontaine, MD, PhD, HDR
Unité de Rythmologie, University Pierre et Marie Curie, La Salpêtrière Hospital, Paris, France

Robert Frank, MD
Unité de Rythmologie, University Pierre et Marie Curie, La Salpêtrière Hospital, Paris, France

Judith Groeneweg, MD
Department of Cardiology, University Medical Center Utrecht and Interuniversity Cardiology Institute of the Netherlands, Utrecht, The Netherlands

Richard Hauer, MD, PhD
Professor of Cardiology, ICIN-Netherlands Heart Institute, Utrecht, The Netherlands

Jean-Louis Hébert, MD
Institut de Cardiologie, Unité de Rythmologie, University Pierre et Marie Curie, La Salpêtrière Hospital, Paris, France

Françoise Hidden-Lucet, MD
Unité de Rythmologie, University Pierre et Marie Curie, La Salpêtrière Hospital, Paris, France

Rajesh Janardhanan, MD
Associate Professor of Medicine and Medical Imaging, Medical Director, Non-Invasive Cardiac Imaging, South Campus, Sarver Heart Center, Tucson, Arizona, USA

Richard Kobza, MD
Head of Department of Cardiology, Luzerner Kantonsspital, Lucerne, Switzerland

Michel Komajda, MD
Professeur de Cardiologie, Unité de Rythmologie, University Pierre et Marie Curie, La Salpêtrière Hospital, Paris, France

Robert Manka, MD
Department of Cardiology, University Heart Center, Zurich, Switzerland

Frank I. Marcus, MD
Department of Cardiology, Sarver Heart Center, University of Arizona Health Science Center, Tucson, Arizona, USA

Argelia Medeiros-Domingo, MD, PhD
Attending Physician, Electrophysiology Department of Cardiology, Inselspital—University Hospital, Bern, Switzerland

Markus Niemann, MD
Department of Cardiology, University Heart Center, Zurich, Switzerland

Florence Porterfield
Department of Medicine, Division of Cardiology, Johns Hopkins University School of Medicine, Baltimore, Maryland, USA

Christian M. Schmied, MD
Department of Cardiology, University Heart Center, Zurich, Switzerland

Felix C. Tanner, MD
Chief Physician Echocardiography, Department of Cardiology, University Heart Center, Zurich, Switzerland

Alessandra Vecchiati, MD
Department of Cardiac, Thoracic and Vascular Sciences, University of Padua, Italy; Department of Cardiology, University Heart Center, Zurich, Switzerland

Thomas Wichter, MD
Professor of Medicine—Cardiology, Director, Department of Cardiology and Angiology, Heart Center Osnabrück—Bad Rothenfelde, Niels-Stensen-Kliniken, Marienhospital Osnabrück, Osnabrück, Germany

Alessandro Zorzi, MD
Department of Cardiac, Thoracic and Vascular Sciences, University of Padua, Italy

Foreword

It has been 12 years since I commissioned Paul Touboul to write a small handbook on arrhythmogenic right ventricular cardiomyopathy. He managed to include almost everything there was to know about this "rare" condition in only a few A5 pages. But now almost everything has changed: the condition is no longer regarded as very rare; it is not confined to the right ventricle; and its management is symptomatic and prognostic and involves much counseling to cope with the genetic basis of the disease. A tremendous amount of research has occurred in this subject, mostly emanating from relatively few major centers that specialize in this disease. In the early 1980s there were no more than 1 or 2 papers a year, but now about 200 publications appear annually.

The editors, Firat Duru and Corinna Brunckhorst from the University Heart Center, Zurich, have reached out to the leaders and senior researchers from these prolific research centers to assemble a complete reference relating to arrhythmogenic right ventricular cardiomyopathy/dysplasia. Fortunately, the editors have enlisted as authors those who first recognized and named the disease, and most of those responsible for the recent advances in this fascinating area. The result is an excellent and comprehensive but very readable text dealing with this increasingly important spectrum of diseases. It is a unique book that should be found on the shelves of everyone who seeks to manage patients with cardiac arrhythmia, because among those who seek advice, there are sure to be patients with this challenging disease.

—A. John Camm, MD, FRCP, FESC, FACC, FAHA
Professor of Clinical Cardiology
St. George's, University of London
Imperial College
London, United Kingdom

Preface

Since the late 1970s, when Guy Fontaine and Frank Marcus first reported their pioneering observations on a previously undescribed disease of the right heart, our knowledge on arrhythmogenic cardiomyopathies has increased remarkably. As challenging as its diagnosis and treatment, even naming the disease has been a matter of controversy. In the early years, the disease was termed *right ventricular dysplasia*, but now the expression *arrhythmogenic right ventricular cardiomyopathy/dysplasia* (ARVC/D) is commonly used, as in the 2010 modified Task Force Criteria.

For clinicians in the field of cardiac arrhythmias, ARVC/D remains a matter of concern because (a) the disease may cause sudden death in an otherwise healthy young individual, particularly during strenuous physical activity; (b) right ventricular outflow tract arrhythmias, which are generally thought to be benign in nature, may be the initial manifestation of an underlying structural disorder; (c) the disease may proceed to varying degrees of right or biventricular heart failure; (d) despite the identification of genetic mutations in about half of the cases, there is significant variation in the phenotypic expression of the disease; and finally, (e) there is not a single diagnostic tool to either diagnose or exclude the presence of this clinical entity. Today, there is a vast amount of evidence suggesting ARVC/D to be a disease of the intercellular junction. Nevertheless, other pathogenetic mechanisms, such as inflammation and apoptosis, may also play a role.

In 2011, we established the Zurich ARVC Program in an attempt to increase awareness for this challenging disease. This program, which is supported by the Georg and Bertha Schwyzer-Winiker Foundation, focuses on providing clinical excellence for the care of these patients and promoting in-depth basic and clinical research for this condition. In this context, we organized the first ARVC/D symposium in May 2012 in Zurich, where international key opinion leaders and national experts participated. This symposium created a platform for exchange of knowledge and initiated various collaborations between different research groups. It was the collective mission of the ARVC/D experts to bring together the cutting-edge information on this disease and print it for distribution to a wider public. The result is a new comprehensive book on ARVC/D with each of the authors contributing a dedicated chapter on their particular area of expertise.

Because the Zurich ARVC/D symposia are planned to be held every 2 years, this book will be regularly updated in an electronic format so that our interested readers can stay abreast of the most recent developments on this challenging disease.

This book includes various chapters on basic and clinical science of ARVC/D. The first chapter describes the fascinating discovery of the disease in detail. Pathophysiology, molecular mechanisms, and genetic background of ARVC/D are presented concisely. Moreover, the mechanisms of disease progression leading to a diversity of disease phenotypes and the challenges in the clinical setting with respect to diagnosis, risk stratification, and therapy of the disease are elucidated.

The ultimate goal of this book is to offer novel insights in all major aspects of this unique disease and to serve as a valuable guide to help readers provide the best possible care for their ARVC/D patients. We hope the book fulfills this purpose and thank the authors for their valuable contributions.

1

Discovery of Right Ventricular Cardiomyopathies

Guy H. Fontaine, MD, PhD, HDR, Robert Frank, MD, Jean-Louis Hébert, MD, Françoise Hidden-Lucet, MD, and Michel Komajda, MD

Introduction

Famed French cardiologist Pierre-Charles Potain said, "Doctors do not discover diseases. Diseases are as old as the world. What doctors discover are small signs previously unnoticed." As the diseases are as old as the world, it was interesting to search the medical literature for unrecognized cases of right ventricular dysplasia. This disease was not recognized because of the small number of cases seen by a single physician, as well as the lack of dissemination of scattered observations on the behavior of the right ventricle.

The chapter that follows describes how the experiences of various physicians and scientists contributed to the gradual recognition of ARVC/D as a specific disease, an entity of itself. Much of the description is written from the point of view of the lead author, Dr. Guy Fontaine, and it is to him that the narrative refers when first-person discussions arise.

The Renaissance

Leonardo da Vinci

During a visit to the Science Museum of London, I saw one of the famous anatomical drawings by Leonardo da Vinci (Figure 1.1). It shows the body of a young woman who died for no apparent cause, since there were no signs suggesting trauma or major organ disease. The unexpected death may have been the reason for the autopsy. Since there were no pathological findings at autopsy, the doctors of Milan, who knew of Leonardo's interest in anatomy, presented him with her exceptional case.

The picture is fascinating. The heart was cut in the horizontal plane, showing clearly the two ventricles separated by the interventricular septum. In other drawings, Leonardo showed a communication between the two ventricles, but on this one plate, there is a perfect anatomical representation of the interventricular

Current Concepts in Arrhythmogenic Right Ventricular Cardiomyopathy/Dysplasia
© 2014 Corinna Brunckhorst and Firat Duru, Editors. Cardiotext Publishing, ISBN: 978-1-935395-92-8

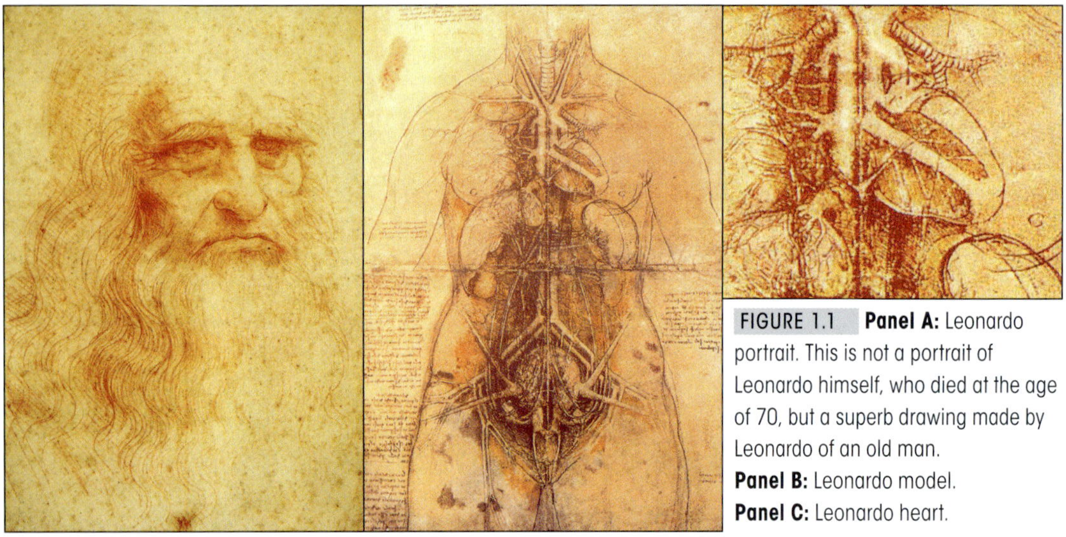

FIGURE 1.1 **Panel A:** Leonardo portrait. This is not a portrait of Leonardo himself, who died at the age of 70, but a superb drawing made by Leonardo of an old man.
Panel B: Leonardo model.
Panel C: Leonardo heart.

septum separating the two cavities. This was contrary to the dogma at that time that physiologic direct communication existed between the two ventricles in the adult. If we focus on the walls of the heart where the epicardium and endocardium are carefully drawn, we can see the configuration of the right ventricle as compared to the left ventricle. The right ventricle is blatantly dilated. The right ventricular wall is much thinner and shows segmental abnormalities. In this anatomical description, it is possible that the patient had arrhythmogenic right ventricular dysplasia (ARVD) that could have led to sudden death.

This anatomical projection by Leonardo can be currently obtained by 4-chamber echocardiography. An echocardiographer who is aware of this disease would assume the diagnosis by looking at the sketch of the master of Milan. The epicardial fat, which is a characteristic of dysplasia, is absent on this drawing. It may have been intentionally removed in order to simplify the drawing, similar to the absence of fat in all the other organs in this picture. Leonardo interpreted the anatomy more as a scientist than as an artist. He sought an obvious anatomical reality leading to the understanding of the physiology rather than making a purely artistic design.

William Harvey (1578–1657)

In Leonardo's time, the mechanism of blood flow was not yet elucidated. Since the heart was known to contract forcefully, it was suspected to drive the blood through the body, and it was known that these contractions were essential to life. However, it was not until William Harvey, a physician from England who resided for several years at the University of Padua, Italy, at the turn of the 17th century, demonstrated the pulmonary and systemic circulation including the arteries, veins, and cardiac chambers so that the human circulation was defined. The French philosopher René Descartes had systematically criticized Harvey's findings based on pure, logical reasoning.[1] Descartes's comments were disturbing to Harvey, and he was forced to make new experiments that resulted in information to the complete satisfaction of Descartes.[2] The result was that the mechanism of blood flow was finally elucidated.

Giovanni Maria Lancisi (1654–1720)

The first clinical description of ARVD was made by the Italian physician Giovanni Maria Lancisi, who was interested in heart aneurysms and reported typical familial cases studied over four generations and one additional family member with autopsy.*

Twentieth Century

Massachusetts General Clinicopathological Exercises (1952)

In the modern era, a comparison of clinical and pathological data as a cause of ARVD was discussed at the Massachusetts General Hospital in 1952. The discussion's chairmen were Dr. Benjamin Castleman, pathologist, and Dr. Howard B. Sprague, clinician.[3] Another participant was Dr. Paul Dudley White. The meeting concerned a 24-year-old woman admitted for abdominal swelling and fever. Ten years earlier, her brother died at the age of 17, one year after the onset of heart failure.

At the age of 20, the patient had experienced 4- to 5-minute episodes of rapid heartbeat associated with discomfort. Clinical examination suggested a dilated heart extending to the anterior axillary line. The rhythm was regular with some extrasystoles and episodes of bigeminy. A week after discharge from Massachusetts General Hospital, she was admitted to Good Samaritan Hospital with acute heart failure. The ECG revealed low voltage with inverted T waves in leads I, II, and III, and in the precordial leads. In addition, she had frequent ventricular extrasystoles. An esophageal lead showed that she had atrial tachycardia at a rate of 220 beats per minute with a ventricular rate of 110. The patient was discharged from the hospital after 3 months, and for the next 14 months, she was confined to her home and had many cardiac consultations. She was treated with cardiotonics, procainamide, and diuretics. During the last few months of her life, she had 2 episodes of palpitations associated with nausea and chest pain. An x-ray taken 3 months before her death showed a right pleural effusion as well as considerable enlargement of the cardiac silhouette. She died at home.

The case discussion was conducted by Dr. Sprague. He stressed the difficulty of diagnosis in this young woman, who had edema in her legs for 11 months, fever, dyspnea, and cough. She died suddenly, but had severe heart failure. Rheumatic fever was excluded, and the possibility of a common congenital disease could not be confirmed. In the discussion, a systemic disease such as von Gierke's was considered. There was no evidence for a collagen vascular disease. The possibility of amyloidosis or granulomatous myocarditis was considered. The most likely diagnosis was myocarditis of unknown etiology, complicated by ventricular tachycardia and possibly pulmonary embolism. However, this did not explain the history of her brother, who died at age 17 due to heart failure. The clinical diagnosis proposed by Dr. Sprague was that of myocarditis of unknown etiology associated with a ventricular ectopic rhythm. The pathological analysis by Dr. Castleman indicated that the patient had extreme dilation of the right side of the heart. This ventricle, and the right atrium as well, were huge and thin, "the thinnest in [his] personal experience." In some areas, the thickness of the ventricular myocardium was no more than a millimeter. Dr. White then asked if there was fibrous tissue, but Dr. Castleman had seen very little, and only around the vessels. The volume of the right ventricle was estimated to be five times that of the left ventricle. In both

Note: A more comprehensive description is reported in Dr. Fontaine's book (in French). It is cited as the last bibliographic reference of this chapter.

chambers, there were small mural thrombi. The valves were normal, and the coronary arteries were not occluded. Dr. White again asked if a literature study had been done to try to diagnose this disease. The only answer was a reference to a heart belonging to the collection of Osler. However, Dr. Castleman insisted that the Osler case was different. In that specimen, both right and left ventricles were "paper thin"; in the present case, the left ventricle was normal in size and thickness both pathologically and on microscopic examination. A congenital disease seemed most likely. In particular, he stressed the absence of signs of myocarditis because there were no inflammatory cells. The septum was also quite normal.

Dr. Sprague concluded that the patient had a congenital heart defect that was not previously described. Dr. Castleman asked if they should propose the term "isolated ectasia of the right ventricle." Dr. Castleman highlighted the presence of concomitant atrial dilation and concluded the presentation.

In my opinion, this was a typical case of ARVD, possibly complicated by healed inflammation leading to right heart failure. The description of the ECG during sinus rhythm was highly suggestive of this disease, with inverted T waves and the presence of both atrial and ventricular arrhythmias that could explain the patient's sudden death. The familial nature of the disease, with the death of a brother at the age of 17, although not sudden, was also in favor of ARVD. The severe dilation of the right ventricle with a thin wall is consistent with this diagnosis. Although the presence of fat was not mentioned, this could have been insignificant. The presence of mural thrombus in the atrium and in the ventricle are well known in patients with late stages of this disease. Dilation of the right atrium can be explained as a result of tricuspid regurgitation due to right ventricular dilation.

Hemodynamics of Certain Cardiomyopathies of the Right Ventricle (1961)

In the 1960s, considerable progress was made in cardiology. It became possible to measure the pressures in various cardiac chambers using catheters introduced in veins and arteries. Variations of these pressures during the cardiac cycle could be recorded on photographic paper, and it became possible to evaluate the hemodynamic status and establish a precise diagnosis and to determine possible surgical interventions.

It then became possible for Dalla Volta et al to evaluate and describe a hemodynamic syndrome called "auricularization of the pressure curves of the right ventricle," observed in two patients with a fibroblastic cardiomyopathy. One patient had a myocardial infarction mainly involving the right ventricle. In the other, the diagnosis was confirmed at autopsy.[4]

This report focused on the consequences produced by incompetence of the right ventricle. The atrium was hemodynamically able to partially replace the function of the failing right ventricle, and the result was the presence of a pressure wave in the right ventricle contemporary with an increase in right atrial pressure. These patients died due to right heart failure, and no arrhythmias were reported. Death was described as "sudden" in one of them.

In a second publication in the French *Journal of Cardiology (Archives des Maladies du Coeur et des Vaisseaux)*, two additional cases were reported. These were classified as "unknown cardiomyopathy" leading to the same hemodynamic syndrome that Dalla Volta established, suggesting a "true clinical entity."[5] These two patients were still alive; however, the diagnosis of one of the patients was not sufficiently established except for the hemodynamic study that was not consistent with dysplasia. The last case is indeed in favor of typical ARVD, since for me the ECG showed obvious prolongation of the QRS complexes in leads V_1 and V_2, an Epsilon wave in V_1, and T-wave inversions in the right precordial leads in a young woman, who is the only one of the four cases to have presented with palpitations (Figure 1.2).

The First Epicardial Mapping in Europe (1971)

In 1968, an abstract reported the first surgical treatment of tachycardia in Wolff-Parkinson-White (WPW) syndrome that was performed at Duke University. I was convinced that this method could be used to treat the most severe cases of ventricular tachycardia resistant to all other forms of treatment including anti-arrhythmic drugs and pacemakers. I recalled a statement of my mentor, Professor Jean Facquet, who indicated that I should not continue to pass the examinations in academic medicine since my accomplishments in the field of cardiac pacemakers were already significant. He suggested that I pursue investigations of "these new techniques that the Americans have and that we do not have." Since I was trained in electrical engineering before studying medicine, and I was convinced that the surgical treatment of the WPW syndrome needed extensive electronic participation during surgery to guide this surgical approach, I discussed this approach with Professor Facquet, who suggested that I meet with the chief of the cardiovascular surgical department, Professor Cabrol, and with his assistant, Professor Gérard Guiraudon. After an interview with Gérard, we decided to work together on this project one afternoon

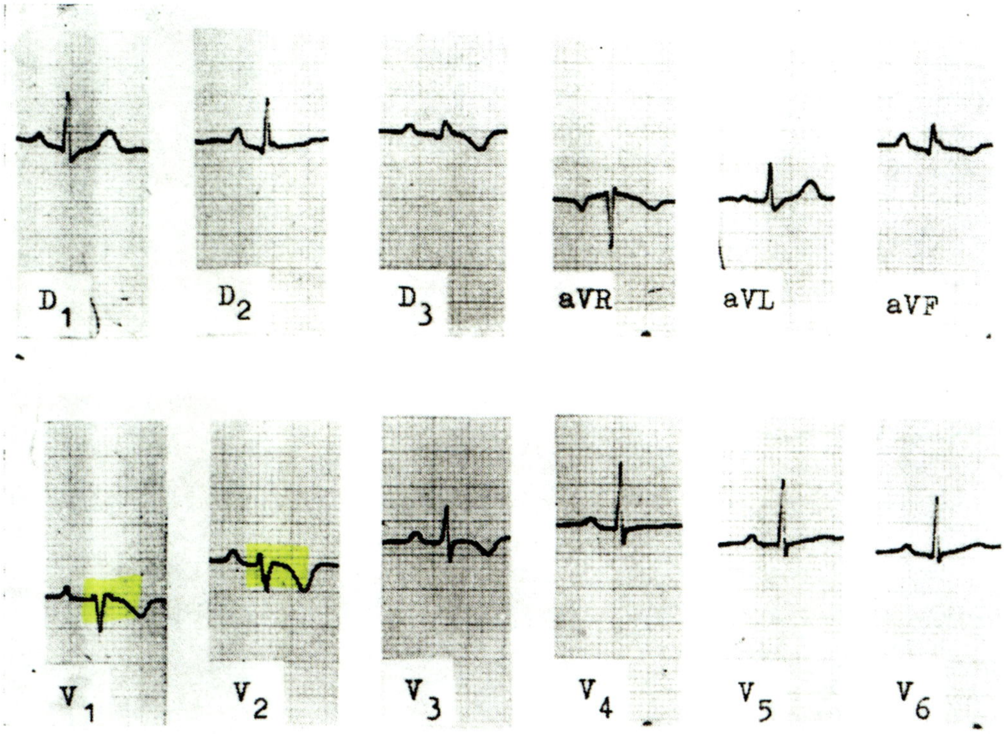

FIG. 5. S.R..., cas n° 4.
E.C.G. : onde P pointue en D_2, aVF, et V_1. Ischémie sous-épicardique transseptale.

FIGURE 1.2 Twelve-lead ECG from Dalla Volta Case Number 4. The comment of the last sentence (in French) is "Transeptal sub-epicardial ischemia."

every week in the department of experimental heart surgery.

After six months, the technique of epicardial mapping was perfected in dogs with a special stimulator that I designed in order to activate the heart and to mimic the various forms of abnormal epicardial activation in the WPW syndrome. We performed the first successful European surgical procedure for the treatment of WPW syndrome in 1971, and a report of this case was published in 1972.[6,7]

It was then that I decided that the same technique of epicardial mapping could be applied to other forms of life-threatening arrhythmias such as ventricular tachycardia (VT). Four patients with VT due to remote myocardial infarction or idiopathic dilated cardiomyopathy were operated on with the same success before we attempted this procedure on the first patient with ARVD.

The First Successful Surgical Treatment of ARVD (1973)

The first patient, a 65-year-old man, did not have coronary artery disease but had had recurring episodes of ventricular tachycardia for 10 years. These episodes were resistant to treatment with all antiarrhythmic drugs. These tachycardias seemed to originate from the right ventricle as judged by the morphology of the ECG during VT. This was of great interest, since VT originated from the left ventricle in the four preceding patients. In addition, the left ventricular contractility was normal, with the exception of a slight anomaly on the anterior wall near the apex. Since the rate of tachycardia was decreased by drug therapy, it could be studied by epicardial mapping. All the documented episodes of VT had the same morphology, suggesting a single area of origin. The surgical procedure took place on October 30, 1973. As soon as the heart was exposed, the surgeon noted that the right ventricle was moderately dilated, hypokinetic, and covered by a prominent layer of fat.

The first epicardial map during sinus rhythm was almost normal (Figure 1.3). The anterior aspect of the right ventricle was activated normally, but with a 10-ms delay. The VT was easily induced by electrical stimulation. Mapping was completed in less than 20 minutes and revealed that the "site of origin" was in the mid-right ventricular free wall as suspected by the electrocardiographic morphology. It was decided to perform a "simple ventriculotomy" along the border of the RV from apex to base. This large incision facilitated an extensive view of the right ventricular cavity, which appeared normal. The histology of the fragment taken from the free wall, studied several years later, was essentially normal with no signs of inflammation. When the ventricle was closed and the extracorporeal circulation was withdrawn, it became clear that the tachycardia was no longer inducible. Subsequently, he had no further arrhythmias and no longer needed antiarrhythmic drugs.

This case was initially considered as "idiopathic tachycardia," and the case report was one of four published in a book chapter after presentation of these cases in 1975 during a scientific meeting in Amsterdam.[8] It was the first time that this innovative surgical treatment for VT was described. Our team was convinced we had discovered a new method of surgical treatment of resistant VT. The patient died at the age of 86 from heart failure without any new episodes of VT.

Left Ventricular Involvement in Right Ventricular Dysplasia (1975)

One of the first ARVD patients operated on for the treatment of VT had a significant delayed electrical activation in the left ventricular epicardium in addition to that in the right ventricle. This was a 42-year-old man referred for VT resistant to all antiarrhythmic drugs. The

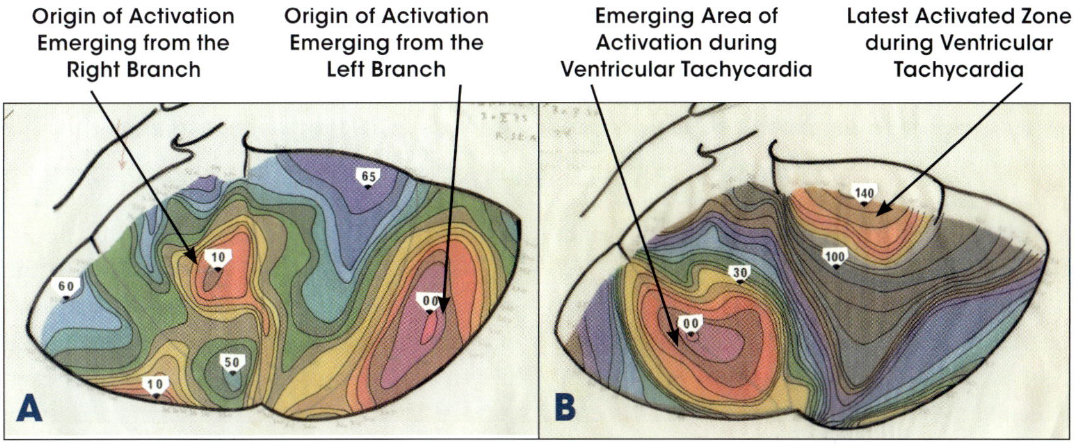

FIGURE 1.3 Epicardial mapping of the first ARVD patient. **Panel A:** Map in sinus rhythm. **Panel B:** Map during ventricular tachycardia.

VTs occurred each month and led to a loss of consciousness. These VTs had the same left bundle branch block morphology, except for some short episodes of nonsustained VT with right bundle branch block observed only after induction by stimulation. Angiography showed akinesia of the left ventricular apex with a discrete area of dyskinesia. The anterior interventricular artery was short, suggesting a probable old thrombosis of this vessel, which could explain the akinesia at the apex of the left ventricle. It could also be due to narrowing of the vessel caused by hypertrophy of the leiomyocytes of this vessel (a well-known feature of ARVD). Surgical therapy for VT was performed on January 7, 1975.

Mapping during sinus rhythm recorded many areas of late potentials at the pulmonary infundibulum and the diaphragmatic surface of the right ventricle, especially at the anterior portion near the apex, but also on the anterior aspect of the left ventricular wall.[9] This was an unexpected finding. It was so unexpected that I rechecked the computer mapping two years later from the saved recordings. I wondered if I had made an error in measurement. However, not only was there no obvious abnormality in any single measurement, but adjacent points followed the same general pattern. This confirmed that there was a markedly delayed area of electrical activity located on the left ventricle. In addition, this location was consistent with the morphology of some bursts of extrasystoles induced by electrical stimulation.

However, during the intervention, mapping was focused on the origin of right VT, triggered by stimulation, and sufficiently stable so that it could be mapped properly. A left ventriculotomy was done as a precaution. It was performed at the critical point observed in the left ventricle based on the information provided by the mapping during sinus rhythm. Although there was a possibility of recurrence, the patient did not have any recurrent VT. After the procedure, the patient's cardiologist stated that the patient showed signs of left ventricular failure without recurrence of the arrhythmias. The patient died 7 years after VT surgery. An autopsy was performed and documented that it was a typical case of biventricular dysplasia.

Naming the Disease: Arrhythmogenic Right Ventricular Dysplasia (1977)

In September 1976, an international meeting was organized in Liège, Belgium. I reported the results of the surgical treatment of VT in 13 patients, of whom 3 had VT originating in the right ventricle. We also saw other patients with VT compatible with an origin from the right ventricle but who did not require surgery. I attempted to classify the patients in different subgroups and found that the patients with VT from the RV had a consistent profile. They were male, young, and had good left ventricular function. They also had VT that could be induced and terminated by electrical stimulation. During sinus rhythm, the ECG showed inversion of T waves in the precordial leads V_1–V_3. In addition, late activation potentials (Epsilon waves) were observed on the epicardium of the three operated cases. At that time, histological data was not available and the electrogenesis of late potentials and Epsilon waves was unknown. However, these were readily explained when the first histologic document became available (Figure 1.4).

I was convinced that a new clinical entity was discovered because these patients did not fit into the description of classical diseases causing VT. I decided to choose a name for this disease that included its prominent features. The term "arrhythmogenic" was obvious, since all patients were referred for the same type of ventricular arrhythmia. Right ventricular involvement was also the salient feature of this group. The last term, "dysplasia," was more difficult to select. At that time, I had no access to histologic material. The only hint of the etiology was the consistently increased amount of fat and decrease in the thickness of the surviving myocardial wall visible when the right ventricle was opened at the time of antiarrhythmic surgery. I concluded that this strange disease could only be the result of a problem in development, and therefore the term "dystrophy" or "dysplasia" appeared to be appropriate. However, because of the young age of the patients, it was probable that the disease started early in life, and therefore the term "dysplasia" was finally chosen.

It was also shown that in some patients, Epsilon waves could be recorded on the surface ECG (Figure 1.5). Finally, the terminology "Arrhythmogenic Right Ventricular Dysplasia" was proposed in 1977.[9]

At that time, I stated, "By an analysis of the data obtained from the operated and non-operated cases, we think it is possible to postulate a syndrome which we would like to

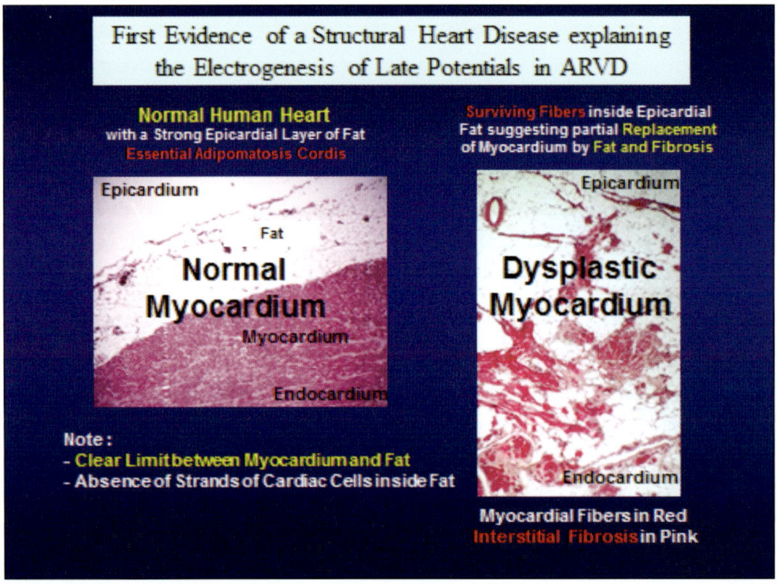

FIGURE 1.4 Histology of normal heart (**left**) and typical ARVD (**right**).

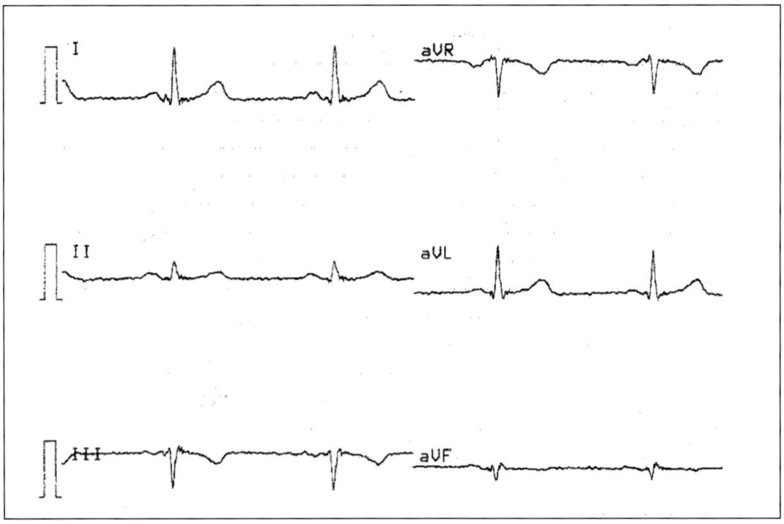

FIGURE 1.5 Overlooked Epsilon waves in the standard leads.

call 'Arrhythmogenic Right Ventricular Dysplasia.' This syndrome may be defined by its main characteristics as follows:

1. Presence of the post-excitation phenomenon, ie, presence of late potentials which can be demonstrated (a) on the right chest leads of the standard ECG; (b) by signal-averaging techniques using digital methods; (c) by intracavitary recordings if the catheter-electrode is close enough to the abnormal region; (d) by epicardial mapping on the thin right ventricular wall. The post-excitation phenomenon may account for some non-specific alterations of the ECG during sinus rhythm.
2. Recognition of episodes of VT with particular features: (a) the QRS complex during VT shows a left ventricular delay; (b) the episodes of VT can be started or interrupted by appropriate electrical stimulation; (c) the site of origin of VT is consistent with abnormalities found at angiocardiography.
3. Presence of abnormalities at angiography. They consist of localized bulges seen in the right infundibular region or irregularities along the ventricular wall, generally observed in the infundibulum of the right ventricle or else in the apical or diaphragmatic portions.
4. Recognition during cardiac surgery of areas of thinning of the right ventricular wall. This thinning may involve the whole right ventricular wall (paper-thin right ventricle), but in most cases, is limited to small areas that appear to be fibrotic and show paradoxical movement."

The Arrhythmogenic Right Ventricular Tachycardia Syndrome (1980)

A manuscript was submitted to the American journal *Cardiology* reporting experience with 17 patients with ARVD, of whom 9 had successful cardiac surgery for VT. However, this article was never published for unknown reasons. Note that dysplasia suggesting a form of cardiomyopathy was included in the first two lines of the text: "We have proposed the terms 'Arrhythmogenic Right Ventricular Dysplasia (ARVD)' to define a particular cardiomyopathy, mainly of the right ventricle associated with little change in myocardial contractility." I later abandoned the term "cardiomyopathy" as being less precise than "dysplasia," which suggests a physiopathogenic mechanism of trouble in development.

Frank Marcus's Sabbatical Year in Paris to Study ARVD (1980)

In 1979, Dr. Frank Marcus from the University of Arizona chose to spend his sabbatical year with me. He was particularly intrigued by the presence of patients with the diagnosis of "arrhythmogenic right ventricular dysplasia," a disease that he had not recognized previously. He was a student of Dr. W. Proctor Harvey, a famous clinician, and he was trained in the classical tradition in the style of Laennec. Therefore, he had the necessary background to study these patients carefully. At that time, we continued to focus on the treatment of rhythm disorders, mostly the most severe forms of chronic VT. In this context, dysplasia appeared as a "disease model." Any knowledge related to this disease could then be transferred to the post-infarction arrhythmias or other clinical entities. All of our activity was therefore directed to VT and its surgical treatment.

During this period, Dr. Marcus was able to thoroughly examine 24 patients with right ventricular dysplasia. He was able to review the medical records and make a thorough study of the literature. He identified a familial case, suggesting that it could be a genetic disease, and introduced the term "triangle of dysplasia" to describe the presence of aneurysmal dilations located in three regions of the right ventricle (infundibulum, apex, and sub-tricuspid region). At the end of his sabbatical, he wrote the publication that is considered the basic description of the disease. This was published in *Circulation* in 1982 and is considered to be a "classic" in the medical literature.[10]

How RV Dysplasia Became RV Cardiomyopathy (1988)

I introduced the term "ARVD" in 1977. At that time, I was unaware of the description of Dr. Henry Uhl from Johns Hopkins Hospital in Baltimore, who at the end of a long discussion was forced to conclude that the strange anomaly he observed on a single pediatric case was probably due to a "trouble in development."[11] The term "ARVC" was introduced in 1988, because it was a disease observed in young patients with sudden death and abnormalities of the RV myocardium of "unknown mechanism."[12]

As I said before, I do not think that the term *cardiomyopathy* was sufficiently specific, because of my long experience in the pathology of patients with ARVD, who showed a very special pathological pattern. This includes:

1. A special topography of lesions from epicardium to endocardium only visible at low magnification (20x), mostly consisting of fatty tissue occupied by strands of surviving myocardial fibers, and endocardium where some fibers were embedded or bordered by a thin or quite thick layer of fibrosis only clearly visible by special staining (Figure 1.3).
2. The same pattern of fibrofatty replacement of the myocardium was also frequently observed in hypertrophied RV trabeculations.
3. It was also observed that the mediomural layers were affected before endocardial and epicardial layers. This aspect was visible in an embryonic case and in some adult samples.[13]
4. The left ventricle was also involved in most of the cases to a lesser extent, showing some areas of fibrofatty replacement, particularly near the apex.
5. In some patients, the same histological pattern was massive, involving both

ventricles, and explained one cause of progression to global heart failure as mentioned above. This was called "biventricular dysplasia."[14]

6. In the late stage of the disease, whitish plaques of hyaline fibrosis independent of the dysplastic areas were visible corresponding to an organized mural thrombus. This stressed the need for anticoagulant therapy at an end stage of the disease.[15]
7. Presence of small vessel disease due to increase in the thickness of leiomyocytes—similar to that seen in hypertrophic cardiomyopathy—was visible in some areas independently of the dysplastic phenomenon.[15] This could possibly explain the atypical chest pain observed in 17% of patients, as observed by Dr. Hugh Calkins on my request (personal communication).
8. Areas of major (replacement) fibrosis suggesting sequelae of a severe form of myocarditis. This suggested the possible involvement of cardiotropic viruses.[16]
9. General overall spectrum of myocarditis ranging from the fulminant form to complete healing with a spectrum of intermediate forms of acute, chronic-active, and chronic with multifocal presentations. Involvement of both ventricles by lymphocytic infiltrations and biventricular failure due to possible cardiotropic viruses explain why two-thirds of these patients die due to congestive heart failure or require heart transplantation.[16]
10. Presence of lymphocytes more frequently observed on the epicardial layers with increased thickness embedding lymphocytes. This infiltration by lymphocytes decreased in intensity toward the endocardium, suggesting the classical pattern of pericarditis-myocarditis, again stressing the role of an environmental factor, probably due to superimposed cardiotropic viruses.[17]
11. Description of the typical pattern of an epithelioid granuloma of cardiac sarcoidosis associated with ARVD, which has been now explained by desmosomal participation in the two diseases.
12. Report of bacterial myocarditis in a typical case of a young adult ARVD patient who died suddenly (while playing soccer). Abscess involving the full thickness of the left ventricle, suggesting that myocardium of ARVD patients is more susceptible to both viral and bacterial infection.
13. Major fatty involvement of RV free wall without fibrosis was an independent abnormal entity called "Fat Dissociation Syndrome."[18,19] It could be a possible cause of irreversible heart failure after cardiac transplantation and has been also reported under the name of "adipositas cordis."[20]
14. Clear understanding of the pathogenesis of Uhl's anomaly, first reported at Johns Hopkins, with total absence of the RV myocardium and apposition of epicardium against endocardium with a small layer of fat in between and the presence of "small vessel disease" in one of my specimens.[11] This disease was suspected by Dr. Thomas James to be representative of an early and severe form of apoptosis as opposed to ARVD due to a more delayed and progressive phenomenon.[21,22] Apoptosis was finally demonstrated by our group for the first time in the human heart.[23] Preservation of a flat layer of myocardium, which explained the impressive delayed potentials observed on the infundibulum of our patient and permitted an almost perfect delineation of the pathway of VT.[9]
15. Discovery of Naxos disease based on typical histologic findings in patients with ventricular arrhythmias originating in the RV with an ECG pattern

stronger than regular ARVD (homozygous nature of Naxos patients).

Discovery of Naxos Disease (1994)

I was convinced that ARVD is a disorder of molecular biology because of my interest in the histology of the disease and extensive review of surgical samples taken at the time of antiarrhythmic surgery (Figure 1.4). The pathology was discussed at length with my associate Dr. Fabrice Fontaliran, a pathologist, during a period of 10 years before we published the first paper on signs of inflammation in hearts in patients with ARVD.

Two doctors from the Greek island of Naxos, a husband and wife team, came to me after studying a severe familial disease with all the typical features of ARVD. In addition, this form was associated with a palmo-plantar skin disorder.[24] The ECGs of these Naxos cases were compared to the ECGs of typical cases of ARVD; the findings were presented in an abstract at the American Heart Association meeting in 1994. This abstract used the term "Naxos disease" for the first time.[25] I recalled the findings of Dr. Marcus and his remark that there was one familial case of ARVD in the original description of this disease, and I was even more convinced that a genetic factor had to be involved in the pathophysiology of ARVD. This led to a decision to approach Dr. William McKenna regarding the possibility of performing genetic studies. The Greek doctor made a trip to London to see Dr. McKenna with whole blood samples from 7 patients with Naxos disease. After 2 years, an abnormality on chromosome 17 was identified, and 3 years later, a mutation in plakoglobin was discovered. A fruitful search for candidate genes associated with ARVD had begun since then.[26-29] The desmosomal genetic discoveries are now well known.

WHO's New Classification of Cardiomyopathies (1996)[30]

When I became aware that Arrhythmogenic Right Ventricular Cardiomyopathy (ARVC) was included in the new classification of cardiomyopathies in 1996, I remembered my previous discussion with Dr. Camerini and realized that ARVC was quite appropriate to incorporate all the multiple facets of the various clinical forms including right ventricular outflow tract (RVOT) VT, Brugada syndrome, biventricular dysplasia, adipositas cordis, Naxos disease, Uhl anomaly, and so on, in which ARVD as described by Dr. Marcus and so on our group in 1982 remained a very frequent form of presentation.[10]

ARVC/D in the 21st Century

How the Term "RV Dysplasia" Was Used or Discussed by Some Experts (2000)

Despite the frequent use of "cardiomyopathy," the term "dysplasia" eventually crept into common use.[31] This interesting phenomenon was initiated by young investigators discovering the disease, the understanding of its genetic background, and the case of a 27-week-old fetus.[32] It became obvious that the disease may be caused by genetically induced trouble in fetal development, and that the original term of dysplasia was appropriate for some forms.

In addition, in 1998, I received a formal invitation from the *Annual Review of Medicine* to write a chapter on this subject. This collection is published each year, and the subjects are selected by top-level clinicians from Stanford and Harvard universities.[33] At the same time, I was also invited by Dr. Hugh Calkins to give a foundation lecture in 2000 at the Grand Rounds of Johns Hopkins Hospital in Baltimore. In the following years, multiple contributions focused on risk stratification of the disease showing its progression to irreversible heart failure in a considerable proportion of patients,[34] the value of contrast angio,[35] and the remodelling of gap junctions as a result of distorted desmosomes.[36]

Dysplasia Controversy and Subsequent Terminology (2005)

Nevertheless, the controversy on terminology did not stop, and is still ongoing. On April 15, 2005, in a meeting conducted by email, Rampazzo (a molecular biologist from Padua, Italy) wrote: "Finally, the name 'dysplasia' was adopted because alterations of myocardial tissue were assumed to occur due to developmental defects. On the contrary, now it is clear that such alterations are the end-stage of a slow degenerative process: therefore the term 'cardiomyopathy' appears more appropriate." Later, the group from Padua adopted the concept of myocardial inflammation and healing as the basis for the disease. For me, a degenerative process or healed inflammation should have produced a right bundle branch block on the surface ECG with reduced amplitudes of the QRS complexes, and not the very small, long-lasting bleeps (called Epsilon waves) seen after a normal QRS complex as has been ascertained in a large proportion of ARVD patients (Figure 1.5).

The International Task Force and the Revised Criteria (2010)

A new period of discomfort came up during the following ARVD meetings, organized to write the new criteria. These new criteria were developed in order to increase diagnostic sensitivity and to identify the disease in family members, in whom the phenotype is generally less severe than in the proband (the first patient identified in a given family). The lack of consistency in terminology was apparent. Each time I had to present my work, I always spoke of ARVD, ignoring the terms used by others, sometimes because it was simply easier to say, and some speakers used both terms in the same speech.

In several of these Task Force meetings, the question of terminology was raised again. An ad hoc session was organized to present arguments for each terminology, followed by a vote. I was the first to speak. After presenting my arguments, for which I had not enough time to prepare, and the comments by the other group members, the final vote was made, giving a slight advantage to the term ARV "cardiomyopathy." At that time, it seemed that the term ARV "dysplasia" was banished forever.

However, when I had to review the final version of a manuscript ready to be sent to *Circulation*, which was in the hands of Dr. Frank Marcus, I stressed again that I definitely wanted to keep the term of the original description made by Dr. McKenna et al in the *British Heart Journal*.[37] Dr. Marcus tried a last time to convince me to accept the term of "cardiomyopathy" and forget "dysplasia." However, after reviewing multiple papers for *Circulation*, I had been selected by Dr. Jim Willerson to become a member of the editorial board for a period of 5 years. Therefore, I was in such a position to say to Frank that if dysplasia was "ablated," I would ask the publisher to withdraw my name from the author list of the revised criteria. In the end, the original term was retained in the Revised 2010 International Task Force Criteria for identification of ARV Cardiomyopathy/Dysplasia (published in *Circulation* and the *European Heart Journal* in 2010).

Please note that the original terminology used for the first description in the *British Heart Journal* in 1994 was ARVD/C,[37] which is the term that I personally always use, but I accepted the term ARVC/D when the concept of multiple facets of ARVCs was my final terminology.

How RV Cardiomyopathy Came Back to the Original Term of Dysplasia (2010)

Now, I would like to give credit to two American experts, one in the field of cardiac arrhythmias who used the term "dysplasia" in the title of one paper,[38] and a second who, after minor criticism by one of the American giants of cardiac pathology, made the statement that "the term, being used for more than 30 years, will be here to stay."[39]

This may explain why, after thoroughly reviewing two manuscripts on ARVD for the *European Heart Journal*, I was asked by the editor-in-chief Thomas Lüscher from the Zurich University Hospital to write an editorial, published as usual in the same issue of the journal. One of the two papers came from the group of Naxos, and therefore I took advantage of this opportunity to give the title "The multiple facets of ARVCs."[40,41] In addition, I received an invitation from an educated writer from the city of Bristol (United Kingdom) to write, for *CardioPulse* (a more social part of the *European Heart Journal*), my biography under the title "Pioneers in Cardiology: Guy Fontaine." This text was beautifully illustrated by the color picture taken with the 5 invited speakers during the opening ceremony of the annual meeting of the American Society of Diseases of the Chest held in Boston in 1989.

Scientists specializing in the biology of inflammation have continued my work.[43] In La Salpêtrière, genetics and molecular biology studies were undertaken; in particular, they demonstrated that ARVD can be the result of a *de novo* mutation. This phenomenon, which is very well known and frequent in the long QT syndrome, may explain, at least in part, why no genetic background can be found in many definitively diagnosed ARVD patients.[44,45]

The Final Consecration of "Arrhythmogenic Right Ventricular Dysplasia" (2013)

It was during the preparation of this chapter that a literature review brought to my attention the publication of an article published in the prestigious journal *Nature*. This journal accepted the use of "Arrhythmogenic Right Ventricular Dysplasia" in the title of an advanced molecular biology article describing using the induced pluripotent stem cells (iPSC) technique to reproduce the disease in vitro using two patients' (from Johns Hopkins) skin samples. Finally, the mechanisms of "trouble in development" were documented with both apoptosis and adipogenesis, both reproduced in vitro from stem cells of these two patients. Therefore, 36 years after its first use in my book, the term "dysplasia" was definitely established.[46]

I will finish this chapter with a final comment on the term "dysplasia," which has not been discussed. During my training at school, I learned Latin, and I was aware of most of the Greek roots of words used in the French language. Therefore, I am obliged to confess that I made a joke in selecting the term "dysplasia" intentionally to see if someone would be, like me, able to critique the construction of this term. Up to this point, the critique hasn't happened. But here's the basis of it: In Latin, "plasia" means "building something." In Greek, "trophein" means "growth of something." Thus, these two terms are equivalent. In Latin, "abnormal" is indicated by the use of "dis," while in Greek the equivalent is "dys."

Therefore, two final valid terms are "dystrophy" if we choose the Greek root, or "displasia," if we choose the Latin one. Strictly speaking, the mixture of Latin with Greek is not recommended! However, as it was said before by Dr. William Roberts, the term "dysplasia" has been used for 30 years and is "probably here to stay," despite being an amalgam of two different root languages.

Addendum 1

Since the first draft of this chapter, I have been surprised by the current problems observed in the proper classification of ARVC patients. Each month we have in La Salpêtriére Hospital a staff meeting presenting all cases observed during the preceding 30-day interval. Between 12 and 20 people of different expertise give their views, until a diagnosis is obtained after final presentation of the contrast angiography, which, at least in our center, remains the gold standard in the identification of different forms of ARVCs.[35] After suspecting the disease based on ventricular arrhythmias, nowadays patients are referred with less obvious signs, such as cases of unexpected sudden death in a family member, and on the other side because of the wide spectrum of ECG abnormalities such as Epsilon waves or Brugada-like ECG patterns. However, in most of these questionable cases with some structural abnormalities seen by contrast angiograms, it is not possible to make a clear diagnosis, and therefore the patients are classified as having "idiopathic" forms of cardiomyopathies. Therefore, it is important, especially for advanced research, to be strict and clear with terminology, and not to put in the same basket patients with different forms of ARVCs, ARVD, and unclear cases of right ventricular cardiomyopathies.[10,42]

Addendum 2

Since the final version of this book manuscript, I authored an important editorial with HS Chen published in the *American Journal of Cardiology*.

> Fontaine G, Chen HS. Arrhythmogenic right ventricular dysplasia back in force. *Am J Cardiol.* 2014;113:1735-1739. doi:10.1016/j.amjcard.2014.03.001. Epub 2014 Mar 14. PubMed PMID: 24792741.

Abbreviations

iPSC induced pluripotent stem cells
VT ventricular tachycardia

References

1. Hurst W, Conti CR, Fye WB. *Profiles in Cardiology.* Mahwah, NJ: Foundation for the Advances in Medicine and Science; 2003.
2. Wright T. *Circulation: William Harvey's Revolutionary Idea.* London: Chatto & Windus; 2012.
3. Massachusetts General Hospital. Weekly clinicopathological exercises: case 38201 cardiac dilatation of right heart, extreme, congenital. *N Engl J Med.* 1952;246:785-790.
4. Dalla Volta S, Battaglia G, Zerbini E. "Auricularization" of right ventricular pressure curve. *Am Heart J.* 1961;61:25-33.
5. Dalla Volta S, Fameli O, Maschio G. The clinical and hemodynamic syndrome of auricularisation of the right ventricle. A propos de 4 cas personnels. *Arch Mal Coeur.* 1965; 58:1129-1143.
6. Fontaine G, Guiraudon G, Vachon JM, et al. Section d'un faisceau de Kent dans un cas de syndrome de Wolff-Parkinson-White de type AB. I-Explorations électrophysiologiques pré-opératoires. *Arch Mal Coeur.* 1972;65:905.
7. Fontaine G, Guiraudon G, Bonnet M, et al. Section d'un faisceau de Kent dans un cas de syndrome de Wolff-Parkinson-White. II-Cartographies épicardiques. *Arch Mal Coeur Vaiss.* 1972;65:925-934.
8. Fontaine G, Guiraudon G, Frank R, Coutte R, Dragodanne C. Epicardial mapping and surgical treatment in 6 cases of resistant ventricular tachycardia not related to coronary artery disease. In: Wellens HJJ, Lie KI, Janse MJ, eds. *The Conduction System of the Heart.* Leiden: Stenfert Kroese Pub.; 1976:545-563.
9. Fontaine G, Guiraudon G, Frank R, et al. Stimulation studies and epicardial mapping in ventricular tachycardia: study of mechanisms and selection for surgery. In: Kulbertus HE, ed. *Reentrant Arrhythmias.* Lancaster, UK: MTP Pub.; 1977:334-350.
10. Marcus FI, Fontaine G, Guiraudon G, et al. Right ventricular dysplasia: a report of 24 cases. *Circulation.* 1982;65:384-399.

11. Uhl HS. A previously undescribed congenital malformation of the heart: almost total absence of the myocardium of the right ventricle. *Bull Johns Hopkins Hosp.* 1952;91:197-205.
12. Thiene G, Nava A, Corrado D, Rossi L, Pennelli N. Right ventricular cardiomyopathy and sudden death in young people. *N Engl J Med.* 1988;318:129-133.
13. Lobo FV, Heggtveit HA, Butany J, Silver MD, Edwards JE. Right ventricular dysplasia: morphological findings in 13 cases. *Can J Cardiol.* 1992;8:261-268.
14. Pinamonti B, Pagnan L, Bussani R, Ricci C, Silvestri F, Camerini F. Right ventricular dysplasia with biventricular involvement. *Circulation.* 1998;98:1943-1945.
15. Fontaine G, Fontaliran F, Lascault G, Aouate P, Tonet J, Frank R. Arrhythmogenic right ventricular dysplasia. In: Zipes DP, Jalife J, eds. *Cardiac Electrophysiology. From Cell to Bedside.* 4th ed. Philadelphia: W.B. Saunders; 2004:754-768.
16. Girard F, Fontaine G, Fontaliran F, Zenati O, Gajdos P. Catastrophic global heart failure in a case of non arrhythmogenic right ventricular dysplasia. *Heart and Vessels.* 1997;12:152-154.
17. Bowles NE, Ni J, Marcus FI, Towbin JA. The detection of cardiotropic viruses in the myocardium of patients with arrhythmogenic right ventricular dysplasia/cardiomyopathy. *J Am Coll Cardiol.* 2002;39:892-895.
18. Fontaine G, Fontaliran F, Zenati O, et al. Fat in the heart. A feature unique to the human species? *Acta Cardiol.* 1999;54:189-194.
19. Burke AP, Farb A, Tashko G, Virmani R. Right ventricular cardiomyopathy and fatty infiltration of the right ventricular myocardium: are they different diseases? *Circulation.* 1998;97:1571-1580.
20. Krishnamani R, Nawgiri RS, Konstam MA, Warner KG, Salomon RN, DeNofrio D. Fatty infiltration of right ventricle (adipositas cordis): an unrecognized cause of early graft failure after cardiac transplantation. *J Heart Lung Transplant.* 2005;24:1143-1145.
21. James TN. Normal and abnormal consequences of apoptosis in the human heart. From postnatal morphogenesis to paroxysmal arrhythmias. *Circulation.* 1994;90:556-573.
22. Runge MS, Stouffer GA, Sheahan RG, Yamamoto S, Tsyplenkova VG, James TN. Morphological patterns of death by myocytes in arrhythmogenic right ventricular dysplasia. *Am J Med Sci.* 2000;320:310-319.
23. Mallat Z, Tedgui A, Fontaliran F, Frank R, Durigon M, Fontaine G. Evidence of apoptosis in arrhythmogenic right ventricular dysplasia. *N Engl J Med.* 1996;335:1190-1196.
24. Protonotarios N, Tsatsopoulou A, Patsourakos P, et al. Cardiac abnormalities in familial palmoplantar keratosis. *Br Heart J.* 1986;56:321-326.
25. Fontaine G, Protonotarios N, Tsatsopoulou A, Tsezana R, Fontaliran F, Frank R. Comparisons between Naxos disease and arrhythmogenic right ventricular dysplasia by electrocardiography and biopsy (Abstract). *Circulation.* 1994;90:I-600.
26. McKoy G, Protonotarios N, Crosby A, et al. Identification of a deletion in plakoglobin in arrhythmogenic right ventricular cardiomyopathy with palmoplantar keratoderma and woolly hair (Naxos disease). *Lancet.* 2000;355:2119-2124.
27. Gerull B, Heuser A, Wichter T, et al. Mutations in the desmosomal protein plakophilin-2 are common in arrhythmogenic right ventricular cardiomyopathy. *Nat Genet.* 2004;36:1162-1164.
28. Pilichou K, Nava A, Basso C, et al. Mutations in desmoglein-2 gene are associated with arrhythmogenic right ventricular cardiomyopathy. *Circulation.* 2006;113:1171-1179.
29. Syrris P, Ward D, Evans A, et al. Arrhythmogenic right ventricular dysplasia/cardiomyopathy associated with mutations in the desmosomal gene desmocollin-2. *Am J Hum Genet.* 2006;79:978-984.
30. Richardson P, McKenna W, Bristow M, et al. Report of the 1995 World Health Organization/International Society and Federation of Cardiology Task Force on the Definition and Classification of Cardiomyopathies. *Circulation.* 1996;93:841-842.

31. Fontaine G, Fornes P, Hebert JL, et al. Ventricular tachycardia in arrhythmogenic right ventricular cardiomyopathies. In: Zipes DP, Jalife J, eds. *Cardiac Electrophysiology. From Cell to Bedside.* 4th ed. Philadelphia: W.B. Saunders; 2004:588-600.
32. Benettoni A, Rustico MA, Fontaliran F. Images in cardiology. Echocardiographic appearances of right ventricular dysplasia in the fetus. *Heart.* 1997;78:200.
33. Fontaine G, Fontaliran F, Hebert JL, et al. Arrhythmogenic right ventricular dysplasia. *Annu Rev Med.* 1999;50:17-35.
34. Hulot JS, Jouven X, Empana JP, Frank R, Fontaine G. Natural history and risk stratification of arrhythmogenic right ventricular dysplasia/cardiomyopathy. *Circulation.* 2004;110:1879-1884.
35. Hebert JL, Chemla D, Gerard O, et al. Angiographic right and left ventricular function in arrhythmogenic right ventricular dysplasia. *Am J Cardiol.* 2004;93:728-733.
36. Kaplan SR, Gard JJ, Protonotarios N, et al. Remodeling of myocyte gap junctions in arrhythmogenic right ventricular cardiomyopathy due to a deletion in plakoglobin (Naxos disease). *Heart Rhythm.* 2004;1:3-11.
37. McKenna WJ, Thiene G, Nava A, et al. Diagnosis of arrhythmogenic right ventricular dysplasia/cardiomyopathy. *Br Heart J.* 1994;71:215-218.
38. Arbelo E, Josephson ME. Ablation of ventricular arrhythmias in arrhythmogenic right ventricular dysplasia. *J Cardiovasc Electrophysiol.* 2010;21:473-486.
39. Roberts WC, Ko JM, Kuiper JJ, Hall SA, Meyer DM. Some previously neglected examples of arrhythmogenic right ventricular dysplasia/cardiomyopathy and frequency of its various reported manifestations. *Am J Cardiol.* 2010;106:268-274.
40. Protonotarios N, Anastasakis A, Antoniades L, et al. Arrhythmogenic right ventricular cardiomyopathy/dysplasia on the basis of the revised diagnostic criteria in affected families with desmosomal mutations. *Eur Heart J.* 2011;32:1097-1104.
41. Fontaine GH. The multiple facets of right ventricular cardiomyopathies. *Eur Heart J.* 2011;32:1049-1051.
42. Kim C, Wong J, Wen J, et al. Studying arrhythmogenic right ventricular dysplasia with patient-specific iPSCs. *Nature.* 2013;494:105-110.
43. Bonny A, Lellouche N, Ditah I, et al. C-reactive protein in arrhythmogenic right ventricular dysplasia/cardiomyopathy and relationship with ventricular tachycardia. *Cardiol Res Pract.* 2010;2010:919783.
44. Fressart V, Duthoit G, Donal E, et al. Desmosomal gene analysis in arrhythmogenic right ventricular dysplasia/cardiomyopathy: spectrum of mutations and clinical impact in practice. *Europace.* 2010;12:861-868.
45. Gandjbakhch E, Fressart V, Bertaux G, et al. Sporadic arrhythmogenic right ventricular cardiomyopathy/dysplasia due to a de novo mutation. *Europace.* 2009;11:379-381.
46. Fontaine GH. *La mort subite du jeune et de l'athlète.* Paris: SFEM Editions Paris; 2010:270-271.

2

Disease Mechanisms in Arrhythmogenic Right Ventricular Cardiomyopathy/Dysplasia: From the Macro- to the Nanoscale

Esperanza Agullo-Pascual, PhD, Marina Cerrone, MD, and Mario Delmar, MD, PhD

Introduction

Arrhythmogenic right ventricular cardiomyopathy/dysplasia (ARVC/D) is an inherited arrhythmogenic disease characterized by progressive dilation and fibrofatty infiltration involving initially the right and then the left ventricles, and by life-threatening arrhythmias causing sudden death. Its prevalence is estimated from 1:2,000 to 1:5,000 in the general population,[1] and it is considered one of the leading causes of unexpected sudden death in young athletes. The natural history of the disease is characterized by a progressive deterioration of cardiac function, usually divided into 4 major stages:[2]

1. **Concealed phase:** Patient is asymptomatic and does not show signs of the disease. However, in this phase, there is a high risk of sudden cardiac death due to ventricular fibrillation.
2. **Overt arrhythmia phase:** Patient fulfills the diagnostic criteria and presents with ventricular arrhythmia(s).
3. **Overt contractile impairment:** Patient exhibits presence of progressive right ventricular disease and initial left ventricular involvement.
4. **End stage:** Patient exhibits severe biventricular impairment.

In this chapter, we will provide a brief review of disease mechanisms in ARVC/D. In the first part, we discuss the hypotheses that have been postulated regarding the molecular mechanisms of the fibrofatty infiltration characteristic of the disease. In the second part, we go in-depth on the mechanisms of arrhythmias. While these two disease processes (fibrofatty infiltration and arrhythmias) intersect at some points (reentry around anatomical obstacles), in others they depart from one another, so that it is possible to see cases in which disruption of ion channel function

 ISBN: 978-1-935395-92-8

may lead to deadly arrhythmias even if the molecular deficiencies are not sufficient to cause major structural damage.

Mechanisms of Fibrofatty Infiltration

The mechanisms of fibrofatty infiltration are poorly understood. The discovery that many cases of ARVC/D are consequent to mutations in desmosomal molecules led to speculation as to the possible relationship between junctional molecules and the regulation of cell transcription. The early studies of the Saffitz group provided evidence of reduced presence of plakoglobin at the intercalated disc.[3-5] Follow-up studies from the Marian lab suggested that the loss of plakoglobin from the intercellular junction may be associated with increased plakoglobin in the nucleus, with concomitant reduction in canonical Wnt/beta-catenin signaling through Tcf/Lef1 transcription factors and consequent expression of adipogenic and fibrogenic genes.[6] A subsequent publication from the same group concluded that adipocytes in ARVC/D may originate from second heart field cardiac progenitors that switch to an adipogenic fate because of suppressed canonical Wnt signaling by nuclear plakoglobin.[7]

While these papers represented a major advance in the field, some questions remained unanswered. Indeed, the cardiac phenotype of the mice, though consistent with a cardiomyopathy, did not completely emulate the anatomical and histological features of ARVC/D. Furthermore, studies in mice lacking plakoglobin show that loss of expression of this protein also causes a cardiomyopathic phenotype. Yet in this case, there is no plakoglobin (nuclear or otherwise) that can lead to suppression of the canonical Wnt pathway.

An alternative hypothesis has recently been proposed,[8] born out of experiments in patient-specific induced pluripotent stem cell–derived cardiomyocytes (iPSC-CMs). These authors proposed that induction of adult-like metabolic energetics and abnormal PPAR-gamma (PPARγ) activation underline the pathogenesis of ARVC/D. However, this study, although highly relevant to the field, should be taken within the limitations of the system. Indeed, lipid droplets were found inside myocytes, a feature distinct from the presence of actual adipocytes, which is the common observation in the heart with ARVC/D. Similarly, no excessive presence of fibroblasts or collagen deposits was documented in this study (these two points suggest that the fibro-adiposis process is myocyte independent). Moreover, several chemicals (some with potential alternative effects) were necessary to induce the phenotype. The authors observed that a chemically induced metabolic challenge caused human PKP2-deficient cells derived in vitro toward the cardiac lineage to accumulate lipids, have increased apoptosis, and present other molecular and functional anomalies consistent with the ARVC/D phenotype. These results are of great importance and potentially revealing to fundamental molecular mechanisms of disease. The data open the door to future experiments where investigators can assess whether the pathognomonic features of the disease can be recapitulated in an experimental system.

A third, much-less-studied hypothesis regarding the origins of the fibrofatty infiltration stems from studies on epicardium-derived cells in vitro. Matthes et al[9] observed that epicardial and epicardium-derived cell cultures obtained from neonatal hearts and lacking PKP2 revealed increased abundance of alpha smooth muscle-actin positive cells, increased abundance of lipid markers, enhanced cell migration velocity, and increased cell proliferation. These studies led to the hypothesis that desmosomal dysfunction in the epicardial cell layer can lead to increased migration, proliferation, and differentiation of epicardium-derived cells, with a consequent increase in the abundance of fibroblasts and adipocytes infiltrating (and in fact replacing) the myocardium. The possible involvement of the epicardial layer of cells is consistent with the common observation that the fibrofatty infiltration progresses from epicardium toward endocardium. Yet the experiments described above are very preliminary, have been done in vitro only, and are still short of validation, at least in an animal model of the disease. On the other hand, the possible involvement of the epicardial layer poses the interesting—if futuristic—hypothesis that gene therapy could be targeted to the epicardium (delivered locally), and in doing so, a local modification of the behavior of the culprit cells could be accomplished.

Overall, there have been major advances in the understanding of the molecular mechanisms of the fibrofatty infiltration characteristic of ARVC/D. The availability of genetically modified animal models, patient-specific iPSCs derived toward the cardiac lineage and potentially toward other cell types (epicardial cells?), and the development of novel molecular tools places the field on the verge of exciting new discoveries that hopefully will bring us closer to a cure.

Mechanisms of Arrhythmias

The mechanisms that cause ventricular arrhythmias in patients with ARVC/D are likely multifactorial, and the substrate varies depending on disease stage. As such, it is reasonable to speculate that the causes of ventricular arrhythmias in the presence of an overt clinical phenotype and structural disease are different from the ones causing ventricular fibrillation and sudden death in the concealed phase, when structural anomalies are not yet detectable. As a gross generalization, one can divide the arrhythmogenic mechanisms as those resulting from alterations in macrostructure (anatomical obstacles, most likely involving areas of fibrofatty infiltration), microstructure (interstitial fibrosis; loss of cell–cell mechanical and electrical coupling), or nanostructure (dysfunction of macromolecular complexes responsible for cellular electrical activity). We state at the outset that these three components are not mutually exclusive, and in fact are likely to coexist in every ARVC/D-affected heart. We make these distinctions as a way of cataloging the various factors that can precipitate the arrhythmic behavior of the patient with ARVC/D.

Macrostructure: Ventricular Arrhythmias in the Presence of Overt Structural Disease

Progressive structural anomalies in ARVC/D, such as regional wall motion anomalies, appearance of ventricular aneurysms, and increased trabeculation, initially localize to the right ventricle (RV) in the majority of cases.[10] Macroreentry related to anatomical obstacles (fibroid and adipose tissue) is the likely mechanism that underlies the arrhythmias detected in this phase of the disease, with similarities to the arrhythmias observed in the postinfarction setting. Indeed, it is generally accepted that the inhomogeneous distribution of fibrofatty tissue and residual myocytes can provide the substrate for slow conduction and nonuniform anisotropy, thus favoring re-excitation.[11] The progressive nature of ARVC/D could explain the existence of multiple reentrant pathways, which predispose patients to recurrences and frequent incessant episodes of arrhythmias, notwithstanding therapeutic interventions. Arrhythmias manifest as episodes of sustained ventricular tachycardia (VT) of RV origin (left bundle branch block with inferior or superior axis morphology), usually tolerated for a long time by the patients, because left ventricular function is still preserved.[11,12]

The anatomical substrate of arrhythmias was recently studied using endocardial voltage mapping, a technique that allows the physician to detect the presence and extension of the electroanatomic scar by identifying myocardial replaced tissue as a low-amplitude signal. In their study, Migliore et al[13] showed that in a population of 69 consecutive ARVC/D patients, the arrhythmic risk was proportional to the extent of RV low-voltage areas detected by endocardial voltage mapping. The authors concluded that the extent of bipolar RV endocardial low-voltage areas was a powerful predictor of arrhythmic outcome, whereas a normal bipolar endocardial voltage map characterized the low-risk subgroup.

The existence of an anatomical substrate provides the basis for a therapeutic approach based on catheter ablation. A recent large study from the investigators of the ARVD Registry[14] evaluated the efficacy of radiofrequency catheter ablation in ARVC/D, with particular focus on novel modalities, including epicardial catheter ablation. The authors concluded that, even though recurrences were common, radiofrequency ablation significantly decreased the burden of VT in ARVC/D patients, with epicardial ablation strategies being associated with longer survival free of VT. Overall, arrhythmias resulting from alterations in the macrostructure represent a group more amenable to diagnosis and treatment, as modern methods of mapping and ablation become available.

Microstructure: Loss of Cell–Cell Continuity, Gap Junctions, and Propagation through the Intercellular Space

ARVC/D and Gap Junctions. Since the discovery that mutations on genes coding for cardiac desmosomal proteins can be responsible for ARVC/D, it has been proposed that defective desmosomes could favor detachment of myocytes at the intercalated discs, especially under mechanical stress, with subsequent myocyte death and fibrofatty replacement.[15] Initial studies by the Saffitz group[3-5] showed a consistent decrease in the immunoreactive levels of plakoglobin at the intercalated disc region of heart sections from ARVC/D-affected patients. Interestingly, the adhesion molecule N-cadherin was not altered, while there was a marked reduction in the gap junction protein Connexin43 (Cx43). Similar results have been also described in an animal model of spontaneous ARVC/D. Indeed, familial ARVC/D and sudden death is a common occurrence in Boxer dogs, which show similar clinical and pathological features as those of the human condition.[16] The characterization of the intercalated disc in this animal model by immunochemistry techniques also showed loss of the gap junction signal among other proteins of the intercalated disc.[17] All these observations suggest that ARVC/D is associated with a significant remodeling of the structures involved in cell–cell communication. In fact, the remodeling of the intercalated disc has been also confirmed by transmission electron microscopy. Endomyocardial biopsies from ARVC/D patients exhibit a decreased number of desmosomes, increased length of desmosomes, and widening of the intercellular gap.[18] Similar results were also obtained in boxer dogs afflicted with ARVC/D. Decreased number of desmosomes, gap junctions, and adherens junctions suggested changes in the macromolecular components of the intercalated disc. Moreover, electron microscopy images also showed loss of cytoskeletal organization in the subsarcolemmal space, suggesting a loss of attachment of the cytoskeletal apparatus to points of cell–cell apposition.[19] Mutations in desmosomal proteins such as desmocollin-2 or desmoglein-2 have also shown a reduction in the content of desmosomal proteins and Cx43[20] and decreased number of desmosomes, while the desmosome gap is increased.[21] Other animal models of desmosomal (or area composita) deficiency have consistently observed changes in the abundance of Cx43 immunoreactive plaques at the cardiac intercalated disc.[22,23]

The Intercellular Cleft as a Part of the Electrical Circuitry at the Intercalated Disc. Together with changes in the abundance of Cx43 immunoreactive protein at the intercalated disc, various investigators have observed a widening of the intercellular gap in both human hearts[18] and the hearts of animals with a desmosomal deficiency.[24] This effect may have an important yet unrecognized importance in arrhythmogenesis. Indeed, new studies have revamped an old idea: that cell–cell propagation of electrical charge does not occur only through gap junctions, but instead, an electric field–mediated transfer of charge can occur between cells. According to this model, the intercellular cleft (and its dimension) is a key component of the cell–cell propagation circuitry. A more detailed explanation of this model is provided below.

Most mathematical models of cardiac action potential propagation assume that gap junctions are the only path for transfer of charge between cells. Accordingly, these models predict that decreases in junctional conductance bring about decreases in conduction velocity. This notion contrasts sharply with actual data showing that only extreme reductions in Cx43 abundance (and electrical coupling) lead to significant changes in conduction velocity.[25-27] These results have given new impetus to the notion that, under poor gap junction–mediated coupling, propagation can be maintained via a separate "electric field mechanism."[28-31] This alternative postulates that the large I_{Na} in the proximal side of an intercellular cleft generates a negative extracellular potential within the cleft, which depolarizes the distal membrane and activates its sodium channels. Thus, propagation can continue downstream in the absence of gap junctions, provided there are (1) a large I_{Na} at the intercalated disc and (2) a narrow intercellular cleft separating the two apposing cells. According to this model, propagation failure in ARVC/D-affected hearts may be consequent not only to the loss of gap junction–mediated coupling but also to the impaired electric field transmission resulting from the widening of the intercellular cleft. Experimental and numerical simulations will be necessary to further assess the latter hypothesis.

The Nanostructure: ARVC/D as a Disease of the Cardiac Connexome. It is well accepted that disruption of the cardiac structure, or of the cardiac histology, can be arrhythmogenic. Yet, lethal arrhythmias often occur during the concealed stage of the disease, prior to overt structural damage.[10] We therefore postulated that mutations in proteins of the desmosome may actually affect the integrity of other molecular complexes, resident in the cardiac intercalated disc, that are relevant for electrical synchrony. Our work has focused primarily on the gap junctions, and the sodium channel complex.

Relationship Between Desmosomal Molecules and Cx43. Based on the elegant studies from the Saffitz laboratory demonstrating loss of gap junction plaques in ARVC/D-affected hearts,[5] we utilized in vitro cell systems to assess the molecular crosstalk between the desmosomal protein PKP2 and the gap junction protein Cx43.[32] Loss of PKP2 expression was achieved by using small interfering (siRNA) technology in neonatal rat ventricular myocytes and epicardium-derived cells. Loss of PKP2 led to a redistribution of Cx43 inside the cell and loss of gap junction plaques, detected by immunofluorescence and also by reduced dye transfer (Lucifer Yellow) between cells. Moreover, pull-down experiments showed that these two proteins form part of a common macromolecular complex that might be relevant to understand the molecular mechanism of ARVC/D. This observation has been confirmed by other following studies looking at the effect of ARVC/D-related PKP2 mutations.[33,34] Furthermore, this complex has been also described to be important in the regulation of the blood-testis barrier.[35]

Desmosomal Molecules and the Sodium Channel Complex: Experimental Systems. A number of experiments have demonstrated that a 50% to 80% loss of Cx43 expression in the heart decreases electrical coupling between cells[36] but does not lead to significant changes in conduction velocity.[25,27] These observations led us to speculate that desmosomes and gap junctions might interact with other molecules that, although not classically considered junctional, also localize to the cell end. In particular, we explored the relationship between PKP2 and the voltage-gated sodium channel (VGSC) complex. Pull-down and coimmunoprecipitation experiments indicated that there is a physical interaction (direct or indirect) between PKP2 and the alpha subunit of the main cardiac sodium channel, $Na_V1.5$. Patch-clamp experiments in isolated adult cardiomyocytes showed that knockdown of PKP2 expression reduced the total sodium current amplitude and caused a negative shift in its steady-state inactivation. Optical mapping in PKP2-deficient NRVMs showed a decreased conduction velocity and a propensity to reentry, in the absence of anatomical obstacles.[37] In a follow-up study, the cytoskeletal adaptor protein ankyrin-G was proposed to partner with desmosomes and gap junction molecules and exert a functional effect on intercellular communication in the heart.[38] Further studies, using mathematical models of cell–cell propagation, revealed that the PKP2-dependent changes in ionic currents were sufficient to induce arrhythmias in a continuous model of cardiac cells, thus emphasizing the fact that PKP2-dependent arrhythmias can occur without changes in either macro- or microstructure.[39] More recently, these observations have been further supported by studies in an animal model of PKP2 haplosufficiency.[24] Mice with only 50% content in PKP2 showed ultrastructural abnormalities (reduced number of desmosomes and increased intercellular space) but not histological or anatomical differences compared to control mice. Furthermore, no changes in the content or localization of proteins such as Cx43, N-cadherin, plakoglobin, or $Na_V1.5$ were seen. However, patch-clamp experiments showed changes indicative of impaired sodium current. Moreover, flecainide challenge in isolated myocytes, Langendorff-perfused hearts, and anesthetized animals showed sodium current reduction, decreased propagation velocity, and altered electrocardiographic parameters larger than in controls. The pharmacological challenge also provoked ventricular arrhythmias and death in PKP2 heterozygous animals, but not in wild-type controls. Separate studies have also shown sodium current deficiency in cells from mice expressing a desmoglein-2 mutation.[40] Overall, experimental cell and animal models strongly support the notion of cross-talk between desmosomal molecules, and the sodium channel complex.

Relationship Between Desmosomal Molecules and the Sodium Channel in the Human Heart. Demonstration of an interaction between the desmosomes and the sodium channel complex in the human heart is more challenging, given the obvious complexities of human research. Unpublished studies from our laboratory, though, strongly support this interaction. Furthermore, immunochemistry studies in samples from ARVC/D patients have also shown that although N-cadherin remains at the membrane, a reduction of $Na_V1.5$ at the intercalated disc can be observed.[41] Separately, Gomes et al reported decreased $Na_V1.5$ at the intercalated disc in samples from patients with desmoplakin mutations.[42] Studies currently in progress are likely to yield new light on these interesting questions.

The Cardiac Connexome. It is worth noting that the relation between PKP2 and the sodium channel complex may be mediated through the effect of PKP2 on Cx43. Indeed, recent studies have shown that loss of expression of the gap junction protein Cx43 leads to a decrease in sodium current amplitude.[43] More recently, Lubkemeier et al demonstrated that a mutation in the C-terminal domain of Cx43 causes severe arrhythmias and, yet, no change in gap junction formation or electrical coupling; instead, the Cx43 mutation drastically alters the sodium current as well as the fast transient outward current.[44]

The results described above led to an important, novel conclusion: Connexin43 is not merely a gap junction protein. Indeed, although a key component of that structure, Cx43 also has some functions that are completely independent from its ability to form gap junctional (or even hemi-) channels. Some of those functions are directly relevant to the proper function of the sodium channel complex. Similarly, PKP2 is not merely a desmosomal molecule. Its presence and structural integrity are necessary for gap junction and sodium channel function, independent of desmosomal formation.

Nanostructure of the Connexome. The functional and biochemical studies described above correlate well with recent data obtained using novel methods that allow detection of protein proximity in the nanoscale. Using proximity ligation assays, the Gourdie laboratory showed that the Cx43 molecules in the periphery of a gap junction plaque (an area dubbed "the perinexus") are not forming gap junction channels, but instead are available for interaction with other molecules in that vicinity.[45] In a follow-up study, these authors proposed that one of the proteins resident in the perinexus is $Na_V1.5$.[46] Separately, our laboratory has used super-resolution microscopy

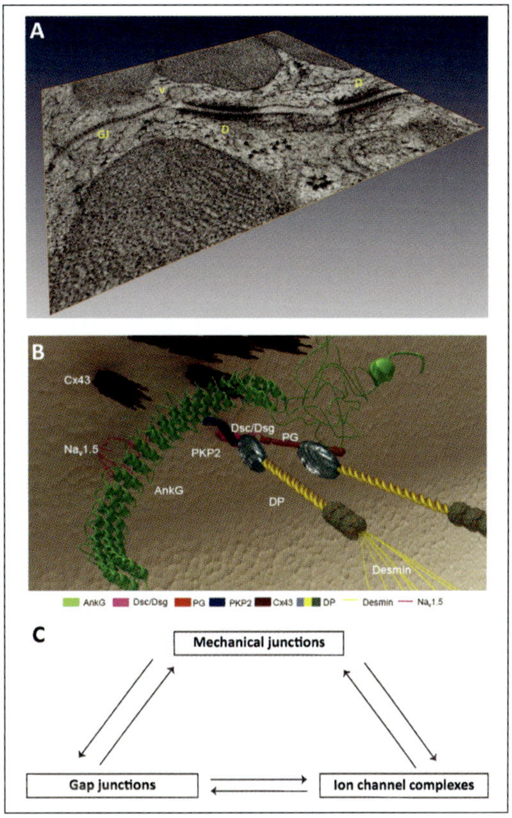

FIGURE 2.1 The connexome: a protein-interacting network that regulates cell adhesion, coupling, and excitability in the heart. **Panel A:** Compiled 3D tomographic electron microscopy reconstruction of an intercalated disc. Notice the proximity between desmosomes and gap junctions and the extensive vesicular activity between these structures. GJ: gap junction plaque; D: desmosomes; V: vesicles formed in the intercellular membrane. *Source:* Reproduced from Delmar M, Liang FX,[48] with permission. **Panel B:** A graphic depiction of the connexome, emphasizing the cross-talk between the different components of the intercalated disc. *Source:* Reproduced from Sato PY et al,[38] with permission. **Panel C:** A diagram of the interactions at the intercalated disc. Gap junctions refer to Cx43; mechanical junctions include desmosomes and adherens junctions; and ion channel complexes refer primarily to the sodium channel complex, although others may also be present. *Source:* Reproduced from Agullo-Pascual E, Delmar M,[49] with permission.

methods (direct stochastic optical reconstruction microscopy, or dSTORM) for the first time to define the proximity between immunoreactive junctional proteins.[47] Our results show that PKP2 often shares a physical space with Cx43, thus indicating that these proteins are able to directly interact and likely regulate the function of the other. The effects of PKP2 mutations on gap junctions and on sodium channel function may result not from a distant effect, but from the loss of direct protein interactions that occur in the perinexal space.

The results described here support the notion that the intercalated disc is the host of multiple molecular complexes capable of interacting with each other. Images of the intercalated disc obtained by modern electron microscopy methods (see Figure 2.1, Panel A) reveal the proximity of these structures and, as such, the likelihood of their mutual interactions. The model of an interacting intercalated disc (Figure 2.1, Panels B and C) is consistent with our results demonstrating PKP2 within the Cx43 plaque (Figure 2.2). Therefore, our dSTORM results[47] and the data from the Gourdie laboratory[46] indicate that PKP2, Cx43, and $Na_V1.5$ populate the perinexus, and that this domain represents the physical space holding the connexome, a protein-interacting network where multiple molecules work together to coordinate excitability, cell coupling, and cell adhesion in the heart.

Conclusion

In summary, we have reviewed current concepts on the possible mechanisms of fibrofatty infiltration and arrhythmias in ARVC/D. Not surprisingly, the global picture is that of a multifactorial disease, where changes in all three scales (macro-, micro-, and nanostructure) are likely to be present, providing multiple substrates for the generation and maintenance of abnormal rhythms. While ablation strategies have advanced the therapeutic approach to patients with macrostructure-based reentry, methods to intervene at the level of the microstructure, or at the level of molecular complexes, remain mostly unavailable. Also critical is the development of strategies to assess arrhythmia risk. ARVC/D is a

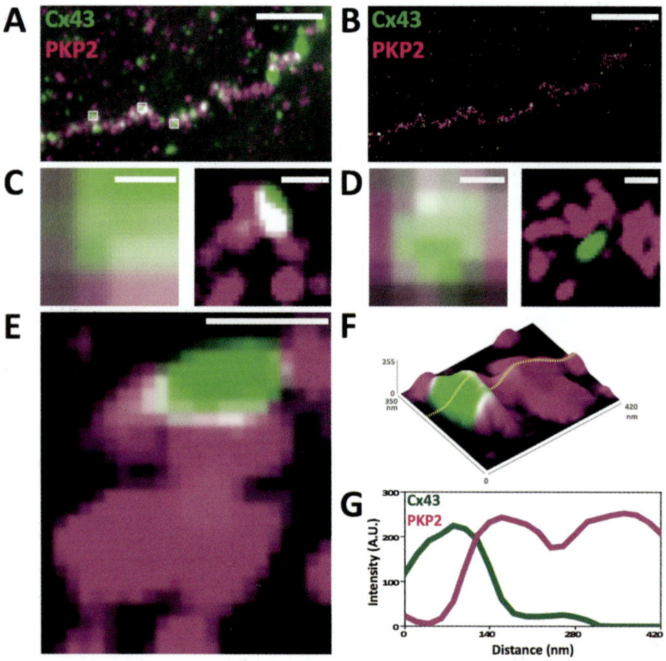

FIGURE 2.2 Direct-stochastic optical reconstruction microscopy (dSTORM) demonstrates the presence of PKP2 (**purple**) in the Cx43 plaque (**green**). For **Panel A** and **left Panels C** and **D:** images obtained from conventional total internal reflection fluorescence (TIRF). **Panel B, right Panels C** and **D:** Same image, via dSTORM, demonstrating improved resolution from ~300 nm to ~20 nm. **Panels E, F,** and **G** show details of the structure of the connexome, with an area of PKP2-Cx43 contact (in **white**). *Source:* For details, see Agullo-Pascual E et al.[47] Reproduced with permission.

low penetrance disease and therefore much work is needed to improve risk stratification and better define the criteria that guide the implantation of defibrillation devices. Improved understanding of mechanisms will hopefully improve novel strategies for assessment of risk.

Abbreviations

NRVM neonatal rat ventricular myocyte
RV right ventricle, right ventricular
VT ventricular tachycardia

References

1. Basso C, Corrado D, Marcus FI, Nava A, Thiene G. Arrhythmogenic right ventricular cardiomyopathy. *Lancet.* 2009;373:1289-1300.
2. Sen-Chowdhry S, Morgan RD, Chambers JC, McKenna WJ. Arrhythmogenic cardiomyopathy: etiology, diagnosis, and treatment. *Annu Rev Med.* 2010;61:233-253.
3. Asimaki A, Tandri H, Huang H, et al. A new diagnostic test for arrhythmogenic right ventricular cardiomyopathy. *N Engl J Med.* 2009;360:1075-1084.
4. Kaplan SR, Gard JJ, Carvajal-Huerta L, Ruiz-Cabezas JC, Thiene G, Saffitz JE. Structural and molecular pathology of the heart in Carvajal syndrome. *Cardiovasc Pathol.* 2004;13:26-32.
5. Kaplan SR, Gard JJ, Protonotarios N, et al. Remodeling of myocyte gap junctions in arrhythmogenic right ventricular cardiomyopathy due to a deletion in plakoglobin (Naxos disease). *Heart Rhythm.* 2004;1:3-11.
6. Garcia-Gras E, Lombardi R, Giocondo MJ, et al. Suppression of canonical Wnt/beta-catenin signaling by nuclear plakoglobin recapitulates phenotype of arrhythmogenic right ventricular cardiomyopathy. *J Clin Invest.* 2006;116:2012-2021.
7. Lombardi R, Dong J, Rodriguez G, et al. Genetic fate mapping identifies second heart field progenitor cells as a source of adipocytes in arrhythmogenic right ventricular cardiomyopathy. *Circ Res.* 2009;104:1076-1084.
8. Kim C, Wong J, Wen J, et al. Studying arrhythmogenic right ventricular dysplasia with patient-specific iPSCs. *Nature.* 2013;494:105-110.
9. Matthes SA, Taffet S, Delmar M. Plakophilin-2 and the migration, differentiation and transformation of cells derived from the epicardium of neonatal rat hearts. *Cell Commun Adhes.* 2011;18:73-84.
10. Delmar M, McKenna WJ. The cardiac desmosome and arrhythmogenic cardiomyopathies: from gene to disease. *Circ Res.* 2010;107:700-714.
11. Corrado D, Basso C, Pilichou K, Thiene G. Molecular biology and clinical management of arrhythmogenic right ventricular cardiomyopathy/dysplasia. *Heart.* 2011;97:530-539.
12. Calkins H. Arrhythmogenic right ventricular dysplasia. *Curr Probl Cardiol.* 2013;38:103-123.
13. Migliore F, Zorzi A, Silvano M, et al. Prognostic value of endocardial voltage mapping in patients with arrhythmogenic right ventricular cardiomyopathy/dysplasia. *Circ Arrhythm Electrophysiol.* 2013;6:167-176.
14. Philips B, Madhavan S, James C, et al. Outcomes of catheter ablation of ventricular tachycardia in arrhythmogenic right ventricular dysplasia/cardiomyopathy. *Circ Arrhythm Electrophysiol.* 2012;5:499-505.
15. Saffitz JE. Dependence of electrical coupling on mechanical coupling in cardiac myocytes: insights gained from cardiomyopathies caused by defects in cell-cell connections. *Ann NY Acad Sci.* 2005;1047:336-344.
16. Basso C, Fox PR, Meurs KM, et al. Arrhythmogenic right ventricular cardiomyopathy causing sudden cardiac death in boxer dogs: a new animal model of human disease. *Circulation.* 2004;109:1180-1185.
17. Oxford EM, Everitt M, Coombs W, et al. Molecular composition of the intercalated disc in a spontaneous canine animal model of arrhythmogenic right ventricular dysplasia/cardiomyopathy. *Heart Rhythm.* 2007;4:1196-1205.
18. Basso C, Czarnowska E, Della Barbera M, et al. Ultrastructural evidence of intercalated disc remodelling in arrhythmogenic right ventricular cardiomyopathy: an electron

microscopy investigation on endomyocardial biopsies. *Eur Heart J.* 2006;27:1847-1854.

19. Oxford EM, Danko CG, Kornreich BG, et al. Ultrastructural changes in cardiac myocytes from Boxer dogs with arrhythmogenic right ventricular cardiomyopathy. *J Vet Cardiol.* 2011;13:101-113.
20. Gehmlich K, Lambiase PD, Asimaki A, et al. A novel desmocollin-2 mutation reveals insights into the molecular link between desmosomes and gap junctions. *Heart Rhythm.* 2011;8:711-718.
21. Pilichou K, Nava A, Basso C, et al. Mutations in desmoglein-2 gene are associated with arrhythmogenic right ventricular cardiomyopathy. *Circulation.* 2006;113:1171-1179.
22. Swope D, Cheng L, Gao E, Li J, Radice GL. Loss of cadherin-binding proteins beta-catenin and plakoglobin in the heart leads to gap junction remodeling and arrhythmogenesis. *Mol Cell Biol.* 2012;32:1056-1067.
23. Li J, Goossens S, van Hengel J, et al. Loss of alphaT-catenin alters the hybrid adhering junctions in the heart and leads to dilated cardiomyopathy and ventricular arrhythmia following acute ischemia. *J Cell Sci.* 2012;125:1058-1067.
24. Cerrone M, Noorman M, Lin X, et al. Sodium current deficit and arrhythmogenesis in a murine model of plakophilin-2 haploinsufficiency. *Cardiovasc Res.* 2012;95(4):460-468.
25. Danik SB, Liu F, Zhang J, et al. Modulation of cardiac gap junction expression and arrhythmic susceptibility. *Circ Res.* 2004;95:1035-1041.
26. Kirchhoff S, Kim JS, Hagendorff A, et al. Abnormal cardiac conduction and morphogenesis in connexin40 and connexin43 double-deficient mice. *Circ Res.* 2000;87:399-405.
27. Morley GE, Vaidya D, Jalife J. Characterization of conduction in the ventricles of normal and heterozygous Cx43 knockout mice using optical mapping. *J Cardiovasc Electrophysiol.* 2000;11:375-377.
28. Kucera JP, Rohr S, Rudy Y. Localization of sodium channels in intercalated disks modulates cardiac conduction. *Circ Res.* 2002;91:1176-1182.
29. Mori Y, Fishman GI, Peskin CS. Ephaptic conduction in a cardiac strand model with 3D electrodiffusion. *Proc Natl Acad Sci USA.* 2008;105:6463-6468.
30. Sperelakis N. An electric field mechanism for transmission of excitation between myocardial cells. *Circ Res.* 2002;91:985-987.
31. Tsumoto K, Ashihara T, Haraguchi R, Nakazawa K, Kurachi Y. Roles of subcellular Na+ channel distributions in the mechanism of cardiac conduction. *Biophys J.* 2011; 100:554-563.
32. Oxford EM, Musa H, Maass K, Coombs W, Taffet SM, Delmar M. Connexin43 remodeling caused by inhibition of plakophilin-2 expression in cardiac cells. *Circ Res.* 2007;101: 703-711.
33. Fidler LM, Wilson GJ, Liu F, et al. Abnormal connexin43 in arrhythmogenic right ventricular cardiomyopathy caused by plakophilin-2 mutations. *J Cell Mol Med.* 2009; 13:4219-4228.
34. Joshi-Mukherjee R, Coombs W, Musa H, Oxford E, Taffet S, Delmar M. Characterization of the molecular phenotype of two arrhythmogenic right ventricular cardiomyopathy (ARVC)-related plakophilin-2 (PKP2) mutations. *Heart Rhythm.* 2008;5:1715-1723.
35. Li MW, Mruk DD, Lee WM, Cheng CY. Connexin 43 and plakophilin-2 as a protein complex that regulates blood-testis barrier dynamics. *Proc Natl Acad Sci USA.* 2009;106:10213-10218.
36. Yao JA, Gutstein DE, Liu F, Fishman GI, Wit AL. Cell coupling between ventricular myocyte pairs from connexin43-deficient murine hearts. *Circ Res.* 2003;93:736-743.
37. Sato PY, Musa H, Coombs W, et al. Loss of plakophilin-2 expression leads to decreased sodium current and slower conduction velocity in cultured cardiac myocytes. *Circ Res.* 2009;105:523-526.
38. Sato PY, Coombs W, Lin X, et al. Interactions between ankyrin-G, plakophilin-2, and connexin43 at the cardiac intercalated disc. *Circ Res.* 2011;109:193-201.
39. Deo M, Sato PY, Musa H, et al. Relative contribution of changes in sodium current

versus intercellular coupling on reentry initiation in 2-dimensional preparations of plakophilin-2-deficient cardiac cells. *Heart Rhythm.* 2011;8:1740-1748.
40. Rizzo S, Lodder EM, Verkerk AO, et al. Intercalated disc abnormalities, reduced Na+ current density and conduction slowing in desmoglein-2 mutant mice prior to cardiomyopathic changes. *Cardiovasc Res.* 2012, doi: 10.1093/cvr/cvs219.
41. Noorman M, Hakim S, Kessler E, et al. Remodeling of the cardiac sodium channel, connexin43, and plakoglobin at the intercalated disk in patients with arrhythmogenic cardiomyopathy. *Heart Rhythm.* 2013;10: 412-419.
42. Gomes J, Finlay M, Ahmed AK, et al. Electrophysiological abnormalities precede overt structural changes in arrhythmogenic right ventricular cardiomyopathy due to mutations in desmoplakin-A combined murine and human study. *Eur Heart J.* 2012;33:1942-1953.
43. Jansen JA, Noorman M, Musa H, et al. Reduced heterogeneous expression of Cx43 results in decreased Navl.5 expression and reduced sodium current that accounts for arrhythmia vulnerability in conditional Cx43 knockout mice. *Heart Rhythm.* 2012;9:600-607.
44. Lubkemeier I, Requardt RP, Lin X, et al. Deletion of the last five C-terminal amino acid residues of connexin43 leads to lethal ventricular arrhythmias in mice without affecting coupling via gap junction channels. *Basic Res Cardiol.* 2013;108:348.
45. Rhett JM, Jourdan J, Gourdie RG. Connexin 43 connexon to gap junction transition is regulated by zonula occludens-1. *Mol Biol Cell.* 2011;22:1516-1528.
46. Rhett JM, Ongstad EL, Jourdan J, Gourdie RG. Cx43 associates with Na(v)1.5 in the cardiomyocyte perinexus. *J Membr Biol.* 2012;245:411-422.
47. Agullo-Pascual E, Reid DA, Keegan S, et al. Super-resolution fluorescence microscopy of the cardiac connexome reveals plakophilin-2 inside the connexin43 plaque. *Cardiovasc Res.* 2013;100:231-240.
48. Delmar M, Liang FX. Connexin43 and the regulation of intercalated disc function. *Heart Rhythm.* 2011;9(5):835-838.
49. Agullo-Pascual E, Delmar M. The noncanonical functions of Cx43 in the heart. *J Membr Biol.* 2012;245:477-482.

3

Genetic Background of Arrhythmogenic Right Ventricular Cardiomyopathy/Dysplasia

Judith Groeneweg, MD, and Richard Hauer, MD, PhD

Introduction

Arrhythmogenic right ventricular cardiomyopathy/dysplasia (ARVC/D) is considered a hereditary disease. Although familial occurrence was recognized since the first report on ARVC/D, only in recent years has the genetic substrate been identified. In 1736, Giovanni Maria Lancisi, the Pope's physician, reported in his book *De Motu Cordis et Aneurysmatibus* on a family of four generations with palpitations, heart failure, right ventricular (RV) dilatation and aneurysms, and sudden death. The first modern, systematic study on ARVC/D in 1982 by Marcus et al[1] also noted the familial occurrence of the disease. Nearly two decades later, the small Greek island of Naxos proved crucial in identification of the genetic basis of the disease. On Naxos, families with a triad of palmoplantar keratoderma, woolly hair, and ARVC/D were studied. In 2000, McKoy et al[2] identified a mutation in the plakoglobin (*JUP*) gene in affected family members.

Naxos disease is a recessive form of ARVC/D. Affected family members have a homozygous 2 base-pair deletion mutation in *JUP*, whereas heterozygous carriers show no sign of disease.[2] Another recessive form of ARVC/D, Carvajal syndrome, is associated with a homozygous mutation in the desmoplakin (*DSP*) gene and is similarly characterized by palmoplantar keratoderma, woolly hair, and typically RV and left ventricular (LV) involvement.[3] Following these first publications on rare recessive forms of ARVC/D, other mutations in desmosomal and non-desmosomal genes have been related to the common form of ARVC/D, which shows an autosomal dominant inheritance pattern with solely cardiac involvement.

Autosomal dominant ARVC/D is characterized by a highly variable clinical expression and reduced penetrance of pathogenic gene mutations.[4,5] Patients with ARVC/D typically present between the second and fourth decade of life with a monomorphic ventricular tachy-

 Cardiotext Publishing, ISBN: 978-1-935395-92-8

cardia (VT). Nonetheless, sudden cardiac death (SCD) can be the first clinical manifestation as well, often occurring as early as adolescence, whereas mutation carriers may also remain without signs and symptoms of disease into old age. This variability, as illustrated by the pedigree in Figure 3.1, may be caused by genetic and environmental factors and poses a great challenge for physicians. Therefore, increasing insight in the genetic background of ARVC/D supports adequate risk stratification and management of ARVC/D patients and their family members.

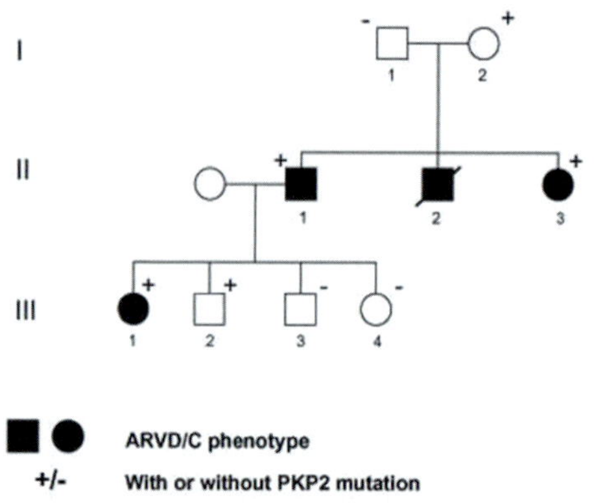

FIGURE 3.1 Pedigree of a family with ARVC/D and the *PKP2* c.1211dupT mutation, illustrating the variable clinical expression and reduced penetrance, which is a characteristic of ARVC/D. The index patient (patient II:1) was analyzed after the sudden cardiac death of his brother at age 17 (patient II:2). The index patient, who was successfully resuscitated after cardiac arrest due to ventricular fibrillation, his sister (patient II:3, with RV aneurysm), and his daughter (patient III:1, with syncope and nonsustained ventricular tachycardia) fulfilled 2010 Task Force Criteria for diagnosis, whereas his mother (I:2) and his son (patient III:2) carry the same mutation but do not show any sign or symptom of ARVC/D. Since the index patient's mother was over 70 years of age, reduced penetrance is clearly demonstrated in this family. *Source:* Cox MGPJ, Hauer RNW. Arrhythmogenic right ventricular dysplasia/cardiomyopathy. In: Baars HF, Doevendans PAFM, and van der Smagt JJ, eds. *Clinical Cardiogenetics.* London, England: Springer Verlag; 2011:82, their Figure 5.3. With kind permission of Springer Science+Business Media.

Desmosomal Genes

The molecular genetic era provided new perception of the hypothesis that ARVC/D is a desmosomal disease resulting from defective adhesion between cardiomyocytes. The first genetic ARVC/D locus was detected in 1994 by Rampazzo et al,[6] followed by the detection of 10 other loci.[7-11] The seminal discovery of the *JUP* mutation in relation to the ARVC/D phenotype directed the search for the genetic substrate to other genes encoding desmosomal proteins. This candidate gene approach identified mutations first in the desmoplakin (*DSP*) gene, and thereafter in the plakophilin-2 (*PKP2*), desmoglein-2 (*DSG2*), and desmocollin-2 (*DSC2*) genes.[12-15]

At present, mutations in the 5 known desmosomal genes (*PKP2, DSP, JUP, DSG2, DSC2*) are found in the majority of (familial) ARVC/D cases.[16-18] In the Netherlands, as in most European countries and North America, mutations are predominantly found in the *PKP2* gene.[4,5,13,17-19] *PKP2* mutations are found in 52% of Dutch ARVC/D index patients and in 90% of familial cases.[18] This high yield of *PKP2* mutations is partly explained by the occurrence of founder mutations in the Netherlands. Haplotype analysis suggested a founder effect of four different *PKP2* mutations.[5] On the other hand, there are geographical differences in the prevalence of ARVC/D-related gene mutations. In Italy, mutations are most frequently found in the *DSP* gene (16%), followed by the *PKP2* (14%) and *DSG2* (10%) genes, which was confirmed in recent studies.[14,20]

Desmosomes are protein complexes located in the intercalated disk that are important for mechanical integrity of adjacent cardiomyocytes (Figure 3.2).[21] Desmosomal dysfunction due to a gene mutation may give rise to loss of mechanical cell–cell adhesion, and leads to downregulation and/or altered distribution of other intercalated disk proteins, that is, gap junction proteins (Connexin43) and sodium channels (Navl.5).[22-24] These alterations give rise to electrical cell–cell uncoupling and slow conduction, respectively, thereby providing a substrate for early activation delay, resulting in ventricular tachyarrhythmia, a hallmark of ARVC/D.[25-29] Presumably, at a later stage, myocyte loss and fibrofatty replacement will have a major effect on tissue architecture, giving rise to zig-zag conduction pathways and load mismatch, further contributing to enhanced activation delay.[30-32]

Although the function of the desmosome and other components of the intercalated disk seem clear, the exact mechanism by which a gene mutation results in the disease remains to be elucidated. Furthermore, not every subject with a mutation and thus a predisposition for ARVC/D develops signs and symptoms of the disease. Additional genetic factors, for example, compound or digenic heterozygosity, or environmental factors such as exercise or viral infection, may explain differences in severity of disease evolution in mutation carriers.[33,34]

Nondesmosomal Genes

In a minority of patients, a nondesmosomal gene mutation is associated with the ARVC/D phenotype. This was first described in an Italian family with a mutation in the cardiac ryanodin receptor (*RYR2*) gene, which is responsible for calcium release from the sarcoplasmic reticulum.[35] Affected subjects had exercise-induced polymorphic VT. Generally, *RYR2* mutations lead to catecholaminergic polymorphic VT without structural abnormalities. The *RYR2* mutation associated with ARVC/D has been advocated to act differently from those in familial polymorphic VT without ARVC/D.[36]

Transforming growth factors β (TGF-βs) regulate the production of extracellular matrix components and modulates expression of genes encoding desmosomal proteins. The gene *TGFβ3* has been mapped to chromosome 14. A mutation in the 5' UTR promoter region of *TGFβ3*, with a predicted inhibitory effect, was found in clinically affected members of one large ARVC/D family. In the same study, an additional 3' UTR mutation in *TGFβ3* was found in an unrelated individual with ARVC/D.[37] These observations implicated that regulatory mutations resulting in overexpression and enhanced activity of *TGFβ3* may lead to fibrosis and thereby contribute to the development of ARVC/D.

A missense mutation in the transmembrane protein 43 (*TMEM43*) gene was found in 15 unrelated ARVC/D families from a genetically isolated population in Newfoundland and caused a fully penetrant, sex-influenced, high-risk form of ARVC/D.[38] The *TMEM43* gene contains the response

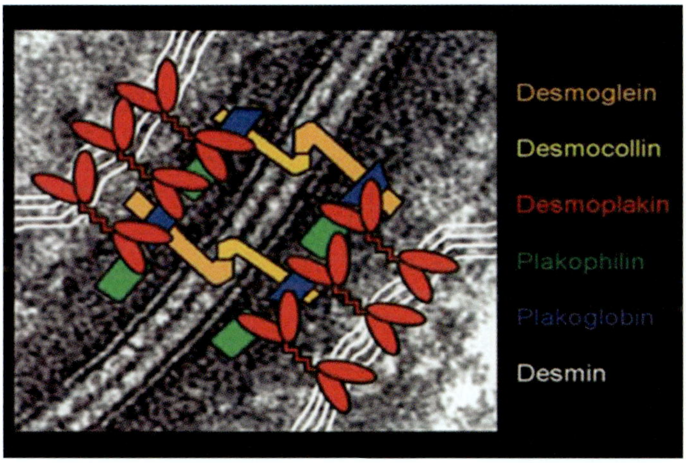

FIGURE 3.2 Graphic depiction of the cardiac desmosomal proteins and their localization. Shown are two cardiomyocytes separated by the intercalated disk. The complex of desmosomal proteins functions as "bridges" between the two adjacent cells, providing mechanical and electrical stability. Desmocollin-2 (**yellow**), desmoglein-2 (**orange**), plakophilin-2 (**green**), plakoglobin (**blue**), desmoplakin (**red**), desmin (**intermediate filament, white**).

element for PPARγ, an adipogenic transcription factor. The mutation is thought to cause dysregulation of an adipogenic pathway regulated by PPARγ, which may explain the fibrofatty replacement in these ARVC/D patients.

Mutations in the desmine (*DES*) gene, encoding an intermediate filament protein, have been described to underlie a heterogeneous disease spectrum with an occasional ARVC/D phenotype. In a family with signs and symptoms of ARVC/D but without mutations in the *PKP2*, *DSP*, *JUP*, *DSG2*, and *DSC2* genes, the *DES* mutation c.1360C > T was identified. This mutation has been demonstrated to affect the localization of DSP and PKP2 in the intercalated disk, suggesting a link between desmosomal and *DES* associated cardiomyopathies.[39,40]

The cardiomyopathy gene titin (*TTN*) was evaluated as a candidate gene because of its proximity to an ARVC/D locus at position 2q32 and the connection of TTN to the transitional junction at intercalated disks. Mutations in the desmosomal genes *PKP2*, *DSP*, *DSG2*, and *DSC2* were excluded. Of the 8 missense *TTN* variants identified in 7 families, 1 (p.Thr2896Ile) showed complete cosegregation with the ARVC/D phenotype in a single large family.[41]

Lamin A/C (*LMNA*) gene mutations were found in 4% of patients (4/108) with borderline or definite ARVC/D diagnosis in a cohort from the United Kingdom, with exclusion of mutations in *PKP2*, *DSP*, *JUP*, *DSG2*, and *DSC2*.[42] These patients mostly had severe structural abnormalities and conduction abnormalities on their ECG. In addition, 2 of 4 patients had classic fibrofatty replacement with endomyocardial biopsy.[42]

A founder mutation in the nondesmosomal phospholamban (*PLN*) gene, involved in calcium homeostasis by interaction with the SERCA-pump, was identified in 15% of Dutch patients diagnosed with dilated cardiomyopathy and in 12% of ARVC/D index patients, in the absence of mutations in the 5 desmosomal genes.[43] Patients with this c.40_42delAGA mutation displayed classic ARVC/D with RV and additional LV involvement and low voltages (< 0.5 mV in standard leads) on their ECG (Figure 3.3). Evidence of pathogenicity was strongly supported by cosegregation analysis in a large family with ARVC/D.[44]

ARVC/D Without Identified Genetic Mutations

Not all forms of ARVC/D are proven genetic. Recent preliminary data indicate that in approximately 30% of Dutch index patients, no mutation can be found by screening of the desmosomal and nondesmosomal candidate genes. In other cohorts, this percentage of proven ARVC/D patients, diagnosed according to internationally consensus-based Task Force Criteria for diagnosis yet without mutations in the known ARVC/D-related genes, is even higher.[16,17,19] These ARVC/D cases may be explained by mutations in genes as yet unknown or by the contribution of genetic variants of unknown significance (VUS) in the known genes. Accordingly, a similar prevalence of familial involvement in probands with and without a mutation in one of the implicated desmosomal genes was found in a study by Quarta et al.[17] However, in the study reported by Cox et al,[18] mutation-carrying relatives have a sixfold increased risk of ARVC/D diagnosis compared to relatives of index patients without identified mutation. The evaluation of a family history of ARVC/D, suggesting an unknown genetic factor, is crucial in ARVC/D patients without identifiable genetic predisposition.

Alternatively, these cases may be due to environmental factors, for example, exercise or myocardial infection. Sports activity, particularly endurance sports, cause volume overload of the right ventricle (RV) and mechanical stress on the cardiomyocytes, especially in the thin-walled RV. In a mouse model with *JUP*

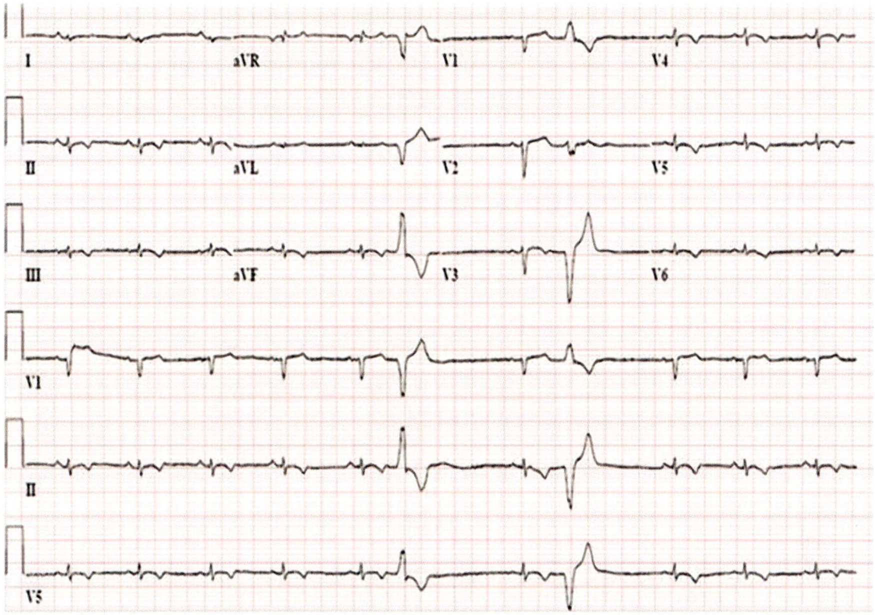

FIGURE 3.3 ECG of a phospholamban mutation carrier (while off medication). The ECG shows low voltages (< 0.5 mV in standard leads) and negative T waves in leads V_4 through V_6 (minor criterion in the 2010 Task Force Criteria for ARVC/D diagnosis). Two premature ventricular complexes are observed, one with left bundle branch block morphology and one with right bundle branch block morphology. This patient fulfilled the Task Force Criteria for ARVC/D. The phospholamban mutation was not taken into account for the diagnostic criteria.

haploinsufficiency, daily performance of exercise (swimming) was a trigger for ventricular arrhythmias and an accelerator for structural RV abnormalities when compared to mice with the same predisposition by *JUP* haploinsufficiency but with a resting lifestyle.[45,46] In addition, in a cohort of 47 athletes (subjects engaged ≥ 3 hours per week in sports with moderate-intense dynamic component, recreationally or competitive, for > 5 years) with RV arrhythmias, excluding idiopathic RV outflow tract VT, the prevalence of desmosomal mutations was relatively low.[47] By screening of all 5 genes—*PKP2, DSP, JUP, DSG2,* and *DSC2*—pathogenic desmosomal mutations were identified in 13% of the total cohort. Of the 24 athletes who fulfilled the 1994 Task Force Criteria for ARVC/D diagnosis,[48] only 4 had a pathogenic desmosomal mutation (17%), which is a lower prevalence when viewed from the perspective of previous reports.[16-20,47] These animal model and athlete studies suggest that exercise is an important contributor to the ARVC/D phenotype, also in the absence of an identifiable genetic predisposition.

Role of Genetic Screening

It is important to realize that the clinical diagnosis of ARVC/D is based exclusively on fulfilment of the diagnostic 2010 Task Force Criteria.[49] Mutations underlying the disease show incomplete penetrance and variable clinical expression.[4,5] Some genetically affected patients may have no signs or symptoms whatsoever, whereas no mutations can be identified in a large minority of clinically diagnosed patients. Therefore, genetic analysis alone cannot be of any critical diagnostic value for the index patient who meets the Task Force Criteria; however, it can be used to identify family members who are predisposed to disease development.

The current strategy for genetic testing in ARVC/D (in the Netherlands) is as follows: Individuals with a clinical diagnosis of ARVC/D are the first to be tested, that is, index patients (probands). The detection of a pathogenic mutation contributes as major criterion in the Task Force Criteria for diagnosis of ARVC/D. However, identification of a pathogenic mutation is not sufficient in the absence of phenotypic criteria. In contrast, if no mutation can be identified in a patient diagnosed with ARVC/D, the clinical diagnosis is still applicable.

If a pathogenic mutation is identified in the index patient, the parents, siblings, and children of this patient can be tested for the mutation via the cascade method. When an asymptomatic relative is found to carry a pathogenic mutation, periodic cardiologic screening is required. DNA analysis by direct sequencing of the desmosomal genes *PKP2*, *DSG2*, *DSC2*, *DSP*, and *JUP* is recommended in ARVC/D patients with an appropriate indication for this analysis. When no mutation is found, this analysis can be extended with gene dosage analysis (MLPA) to detect larger deletion or insertion mutations and with the screening of nondesmosomal genes (*RYR2*, *TGFβ3*, *TMEM43*, *DES*, *TTN*, *LMNA*, and *PLN*). Nondesmosomal genes can be screened according to their geographical prevalence or according to the observed phenotype. For example, in the presence of low voltages on the ECG, *PLN* screening can be performed, while conduction disorders could be suggestive of *LMNA* mutations.

Genetic analysis in ARVC/D at present is performed with the candidate gene approach. However, the development of new techniques for genetic screening is rapidly progressing. One of those new techniques is analysis by next-generation sequencing. With this technique, the analysis is faster and it permits analysis of larger numbers of genes compared to the candidate gene approach. This might result in the discovery of new ARVC/D-related genes. On the other hand, the findings of associated large numbers of genetic VUS will also result in more uncertainty for the patient, family members, and the physician.

Interpretation of Genetic Screening

The interpretation of the outcome of molecular genetic screening in ARVC/D index patients can be challenging. Screening might result in the finding of (1) proven pathogenic mutations, (2) most likely pathogenic mutations, (3) VUS, (4) polymorphisms, or (5) no abnormalities compared to control populations. An overview of the proven pathogenic and most likely pathogenic mutations identified in Dutch ARVC/D index patients is shown in Table 3.1.

The pathogenicity of radical mutations—that is, truncating or splice site mutations (mutations affecting the invariant AG splice-acceptor and GU splice-donor sites of exons) resulting in truncation or absence of the protein product from the mutated allele—is widely accepted (proven pathogenic). However, the pathogenicity of missense variants (also known as nonsynonymous single nucleotide variants) resulting in a single amino acid substitution is more difficult to delineate. As with other clinical tests, understanding of the extent and spectrum of genetic variation in the healthy population is necessary for correct interpretation.

TABLE 3.1 Mutations identified in Dutch ARVC/D index patients

GENE	NUCLEOTIDE CHANGE	AMINO ACID CHANGE	MUTATION TYPE
	PROVEN PATHOGENIC MUTATIONS		
PKP2	deletion exons 1-4	p.(?)	deletion
	deletion exons 8-14	p.(?)	deletion
	deletion exons 1-14	p.(?)	deletion
	deletion exon 8	p.(?)	deletion
	deletion exon 10	p.(?)	deletion
	c.148_151del	p.(Thr50fs)	frameshift
	c.235C > T	p.(Arg79*)	nonsense
	c.258T > G	p.(Tyr86*)	nonsense
	c.397C > T	p.(Gln133*)	nonsense
	c.917_918del	p.(Pro318fs)	frameshift
	c.968_971del	p.(Gln323fs)	frameshift
	c.1211dup	p.(Val406fs)	frameshift
	c.1237C > T	p.(Arg413*)	nonsense
	c.1369_1372del	p.(Gln457*)	nonsense
	c.1378G > A	p.(Val445fs) #	frameshift
	c.1511-2A > G	p.(?)	splice site
	c.1848C > A	p.(Tyr616*)	nonsense
	c.1951C > T	p.(Arg651*)	nonsense
	c.2028G > A	p.(Trp676*)	nonsense
	c.2034G > A	p.(Trp678*)	nonsense
	c.2146-1G > C	p.(Met716fs) #	frameshift
	c.2386T > C	p.(Cys796Arg)	missense
	c.2421C > A	p.(Tyr807*)	nonsense
	c.2489+1G > A	p.(Lys768fs) #	frameshift
	c.2489+4A > C	p.(Lys768fs) #	frameshift
	c.2509del	p.(Ser837fs)	frameshift
	c.2544G > A	p.(Trp848*)	nonsense
	c.2554delG	p.(Glu852fs)	frameshift
DSP	c.3337C > T	p.(Arg1113*)	nonsense
	c.5419C > T	p.(Gln1807*)	nonsense
DSG2	c.378+2T > G	p.(?)	splice site
DSC2	c.942+3A > G	p.(?)	splice site
	c.943-1G > A	p.(?)	splice site
PLN	c.40_42del	p.(Arg14*)	nonsense
	MOST LIKELY PATHOGENIC MUTATIONS		
PKP2	c.1844C > T	p.(Ser615Phe)	missense
	c.2062T > C	p.(Ser688Pro)	missense
	c.2615C > T	p.(Thr872Ile)	missense
DSP	c.1982A > T	p.(Asn661Ile)	missense
	c.6881C > G	p.(Ala2294Gly)	missense
DSG2	c.137G > A	p.(Arg46Gln)	missense
	c.614C > T	p.(Pro2015Leu)	missense
	c.874C > T	p.(Arg292Cys)	missense
	c.889G > A	p.(Asp297Asn)	missense
	c.1072G > A	p.(Ala358Thr)	missense

GENE	NUCLEOTIDE CHANGE	AMINO ACID CHANGE	MUTATION TYPE
DSC2	c.608G > A	p.(Arg203His)	missense
TMEM43	c.718C > T	p.(Arg240Cys)	missense

Proven pathogenic mutations, that is, truncating (deletion, frameshift, nonsense) and splice site mutations, and most likely pathogenic mutations identified in ARVC/D index patients in the Netherlands. Missense mutations were considered most likely pathogenic mutations when (1) predictive algorithms SIFT and PolyPhen-2 predicted pathogenicity (SIFT < 0.02, PolyPhen-2 > 0.900) and (2) mutations were rare in the general population (minor allele frequency ≤ 0.05% in ESP exome dataset). #: RNA experiments by our group showed that this nucleotide substitution leads to the use of a cryptic splice site and results in a frameshift (c.1378G > A r.1333_1378del p.(Val445fs)), (c.2146-1G > C r.2146_2299del p.(Met716fs)), and (c.2489+4A > C r.2300_2489del p.(Lys768fs)), manuscript in preparation.

In the study by Kapplinger et al,[50] the results of molecular genetic analysis were compared between 175 proven ARVC/D cases and a control population of 427 unrelated, ostensibly healthy individuals. Of the ARVC/D cases, 58% hosted a genetic variation that met criteria of a mutation (variation predicted to alter the protein) versus 16% of healthy controls. Radical mutations were significantly more prevalent in the proven ARVC/D cases than in controls (49.9% versus 0.47%, $P < 9.8 \times 10^{-44}$), confirming the accepted assumption of pathogenicity.[50] However, missense variants were found at similar rates in cases and controls. Three associations were identified, which might strengthen the pathogenicity of missense variants found: (1) a rare missense variant identified in a Caucasian patient is more likely to be pathogenic than in a non-Caucasian patient; (2) specific amino-terminal regions in *DSP* and *DSG2* contain mutation "hot-spots"; and (3) missense variants that involve a highly conserved residue in *PKP2* and *DSG2* are more likely to be pathogenic.[50] Most likely pathogenicity of specific missense mutations is supported by predictive algorithms, such as SIFT and PolyPhen-2.

When properly interpreted, molecular genetic analysis allows ultimately the early detection of presymptomatic disease, identification of individuals at risk, and genetic counseling for this sudden death-predisposing disease. Nonetheless, regardless of the suggestion of pathogenicity of an identified mutation, genetic analysis results should be viewed as probabilistic and as part of the overall clinical assessment.

Genotype–Phenotype Correlation Analysis

The identification of a pathogenic mutation distinguishes individuals with a predisposition for ARVC/D. This is a first step in risk stratification of ARVC/D index patients and family members. Nevertheless, one of the primary therapeutic goals is timely diagnosis of the "concealed phase," when individuals are at risk for arrhythmias despite absence of symptoms. Genotype–phenotype correlation analysis can provide more insight in risk profiles of index patients and family members. Most genotype–phenotype correlation studies focused on overt index patients.[4,5,16,19,20,51-53] Yet, index patients are by definition affected by the disease. Therefore, the effect of the genotype can be more objectively assessed in family members who provide the opportunity of prospective follow-up from a young age.

In a genotype–phenotype study by Quarta et al[17] including both ARVC/D index patients and family members, it was shown that SCD was the presenting symptom in half of the index patients. SCD occurred in 31% at young age, between 14 and 20 years, confirming that adolescence is a vulnerable period for fatal ventricular arrhythmias in ARVC/D. In contrast to index patients, mutation-positive family members had a better prognosis, with signs and symptoms of ARVC/D present in 50% of relatives in their fifth decade of life.[17] The differences between index patients who presented with SCD and relatives with milder disease expression may be explained by the presence of multiple versus single genetic variants. Accordingly, family members with more than one genetic variant had a significant (fivefold) increase in risk of disease expression, providing further evidence of gene–gene interactions and gene–dose effects.[17]

A genotype–phenotype follow-up study of ARVC/D index patients and family members by our group showed that a pathogenic mutation in an index patient predicts outcome in family members.[18] Pathogenic desmosomal mutations were identified in 58% of index patients, predominantly truncating *PKP2* mutations (78%). The study included 302 family members, of whom 137 carried pathogenic and most likely pathogenic mutations. Compared to relatives of index patients without mutations, mutation-carrying family members had (1) a sixfold risk of ARVC/D diagnosis, (2) a markedly enhanced risk for ventricular arrhythmias, and (3) earlier onset of ARVC/D signs and symptoms.[18] In young relatives (below the age of 20 years), SCD and other signs of ARVC/D occurred in *PKP2* mutation carriers.[18] Diagnosis of ARVC/D was made in 39% of mutation-carrying family members with a comparable one-third of mutation-positive relatives with a definite ARVC/D diagnosis found in the study by Quarta et al.[17,18]

Although of great importance for risk stratification in ARVC/D, genotype–phenotype correlation studies are generally hampered by the small number of patients and family members. Rare genetic variants are found infrequently. Therefore, large numbers of patients and relatives per specific variant are needed to assess its contribution to the ARVC/D phenotype. Large numbers of family members are also needed to assess variability of disease expression within a family by genetic modifiers or environmental factors. Future studies will be required to elaborate further on risk stratification by genotype–phenotype correlation analysis.

Acknowledgments

We thank Dr. Dennis Dooijes for critical review of this chapter.

Abbreviations

LV	left ventricle, left ventricular
RV	right ventricle, right ventricular
SCD	sudden cardiac death
VT	ventricular tachycardia

References

1. Marcus FI, Fontaine GH, Guiraudon G, et al. Right ventricular dysplasia: a report of 24 adult cases. *Circulation.* 1982;65:384-398.
2. McKoy G, Protonotarios N, Crosby A, et al. Identification of a deletion in plakoglobin in arrhythmogenic right ventricular cardiomyopathy with palmoplantar keratoderma and woolly hair (Naxos disease). *Lancet.* 2000;355:2119-2124.
3. Norgett EE, Hatsell SJ, Carvajal-Huerta L, et al. Recessive mutation in desmoplakin disrupts desmoplakin-intermediate filament interactions and causes dilated cardiomyopathy, woolly hair and keratoderma. *Hum Mol Genet.* 2000;9:2761-2766.
4. Dalal D, Molin LH, Piccini J, et al. Clinical features of arrhythmogenic right ventricular dysplasia/cardiomyopathy associated with mutations in plakophilin-2. *Circulation.* 2006;113:1641-1649.
5. van Tintelen JP, Entius MM, Bhuiyan ZA, et al. Plakophilin-2 mutations are the major determinant of familial arrhythmogenic right ventricular dysplasia/cardiomyopathy. *Circulation.* 2006;113:1650-1658.
6. Rampazzo A, Nava A, Danieli GA, et al. The gene for arrhythmogenic right ventricular cardiomyopathy maps to chromosome 14q23-q24. *Hum Mol Genet.* 1994;3:959-962.

7. Rampazzo A, Nava A, Miorin M, et al. ARVD4, a new locus for arrhythmogenic right ventricular cardiomyopathy, maps to chromosome 2 long arm. *Genomics.* 1997;45:259-263.
8. Ahmad F, Li D, Karibe A, et al. Localization of a gene responsible for arrhythmogenic right ventricular dysplasia to chromosome 3p23. *Circulation.* 1998;98: 2791-2795.
9. Li D, Ahmad F, Gardner MJ, et al. The locus of a novel gene responsible for arrhythmogenic right-ventricular dysplasia characterized by early onset and high penetrance maps to chromosome 10p12-p14. *Am J Hum Genet.* 2000;66:148-156.
10. Melberg A, Oldfors A, Blomstrom-Lundqvist C, et al. Autosomal dominant myofibrillar myopathy with arrhythmogenic right ventricular cardiomyopathy linked to chromosome 10q. *Ann Neurol.* 1999;46:684-692.
11. Severini GM, Krajinovic M, Pinamonti B, et al. A new locus for arrhythmogenic right ventricular dysplasia on the long arm of chromosome 14. *Genomics.* 1996;31:193-200.
12. Rampazzo A, Nava A, Malacrida S, et al. Mutation in human desmoplakin domain binding to plakoglobin causes a dominant form of arrhythmogenic right ventricular cardiomyopathy. *Am J Hum Genet.* 2002;71:1200-1206.
13. Gerull B, Heuser A, Wichter T, et al. Mutations in the desmosomal protein plakophilin-2 are common in arrhythmogenic right ventricular cardiomyopathy. *Nat Genet.* 2004;36:1162-1164.
14. Pilichou K, Nava A, Basso C, et al. Mutations in desmoglein-2 gene are associated with arrhythmogenic right ventricular cardiomyopathy. *Circulation.* 2006;113:1171-1179.
15. Syrris P, Ward D, Evans A, et al. Arrhythmogenic right ventricular dysplasia/cardiomyopathy associated with mutations in the desmosomal gene desmocollin-2. *Am J Hum Genet.* 2006;79:978-984.
16. den Haan AD, Tan BY, Zikusoka MN, et al. Comprehensive desmosome mutation analysis in North Americans with arrhythmogenic right ventricular dysplasia/cardiomyopathy. *Circ Cardiovasc Genet.* 2009;2:428-435.
17. Quarta G, Muir A, Pantazis A, et al. Familial evaluation in arrhythmogenic right ventricular cardiomyopathy: impact of genetics and revised Task Force Criteria. *Circulation.* 2011;123:2701-2709.
18. Cox MG, van der Zwaag PA, van der Werf C, et al. Arrhythmogenic right ventricular dysplasia/cardiomyopathy: pathogenic desmosome mutations in index-patients predict outcome of family screening: Dutch arrhythmogenic right ventricular dysplasia/cardiomyopathy genotype–phenotype follow-up study. *Circulation.* 2011;123:2690-2700.
19. Fressart V, Duthoit G, Donal E, et al. Desmosomal gene analysis in arrhythmogenic right ventricular dysplasia/cardiomyopathy: spectrum of mutations and clinical impact in practice. *Europace.* 2010;12:861-868.
20. Bauce B, Nava A, Beffagna G, et al. Multiple mutations in desmosomal proteins encoding genes in arrhythmogenic right ventricular cardiomyopathy/dysplasia. *Heart Rhythm.* 2010;7:22-29.
21. Kaplan SR, Gard JJ, Carvajal-Huerta L, Ruiz-Cabezas JC, Thiene G, Saffitz JE. Structural and molecular pathology of the heart in Carvajal syndrome. *Cardiovasc Pathol.* 2004;13:26-32.
22. Oxford EM, Musa H, Maass K, Coombs W, Taffet SM, Delmar M. Connexin43 remodeling caused by inhibition of plakophilin-2 expression in cardiac cells. *Circ Res.* 2007;101:703-711.
23. Sato PY, Musa H, Coombs W, et al. Loss of plakophilin-2 expression leads to decreased sodium current and slower conduction velocity in cultured cardiac myocytes. *Circ Res.* 2009;105:523-526.
24. Noorman M, van der Heyden MA, van Veen TA, et al. Cardiac cell-cell junctions in health and disease: electrical versus mechanical coupling. *J Mol Cell Cardiol.* 2009;47:23-31.
25. Saffitz JE. Dependence of electrical coupling on mechanical coupling in cardiac myocytes: insights gained from cardiomyopathies caused by defects in cell-cell connections. *Ann NY Acad Sci.* 2005;1047:336-344.
26. Garcia-Gras E, Lombardi R, Giocondo MJ, et al. Suppression of canonical Wnt/beta-

catenin signaling by nuclear plakoglobin recapitulates phenotype of arrhythmogenic right ventricular cardiomyopathy. *J Clin Invest.* 2006;116:2012-2021.
27. Basso C, Czarnowska E, Della Barbera M, et al. Ultrastructural evidence of intercalated disc remodelling in arrhythmogenic right ventricular cardiomyopathy: an electron microscopy investigation on endomyocardial biopsies. *Eur Heart J.* 2006;27:1847-1854.
28. Asimaki A, Tandri H, Huang H, et al. A new diagnostic test for arrhythmogenic right ventricular cardiomyopathy. *N Engl J Med.* 2009;360:1075-1084.
29. Cerrone M, Noorman M, Lin X, et al. Sodium current deficit and arrhythmogenesis in a murine model of plakophilin-2 haploinsufficiency. *Cardiovasc Res.* 2012;95:460-468.
30. de Bakker JM, van Capelle FJ, Janse MJ, et al. Slow conduction in the infarcted human heart. "Zigzag" course of activation. *Circulation.* 1993;88:915-926.
31. Cabo C, Pertsov AM, Baxter WT, Davidenko JM, Gray RA, Jalife J. Wave-front curvature as a cause of slow conduction and block in isolated cardiac muscle. *Circ Res.* 1994;75:1014-1028.
32. Ellison KE, Friedman PL, Ganz LI, Stevenson WG. Entrainment mapping and radiofrequency catheter ablation of ventricular tachycardia in right ventricular dysplasia. *J Am Coll Cardiol.* 1998;32:724-728.
33. Xu T, Yang Z, Vatta M, et al, Multidisciplinary Study of Right Ventricular Dysplasia Investigators. Compound and digenic heterozygosity contributes to arrhythmogenic right ventricular cardiomyopathy. *J Am Coll Cardiol.* 2010;55:587-597.
34. Sen-Chowdhry S, Syrris P, Pantazis A, Quarta G, McKenna WJ, Chambers JC. Mutational heterogeneity, modifier genes, and environmental influences contribute to phenotypic diversity of arrhythmogenic cardiomyopathy. *Circ Cardiovasc Genet.* 2010;3:323-330.
35. Tiso N, Stephan DA, Nava A, et al. Identification of mutations in the cardiac ryanodine receptor gene in families affected with arrhythmogenic right ventricular cardiomyopathy type 2 (ARVD2). *Hum Mol Genet.* 2001;10:189-194.
36. Tiso N, Salamon M, Bagattin A, Danieli GA, Argenton F, Bortolussi M. The binding of the RyR2 calcium channel to its gating protein FKBP12.6 is oppositely affected by ARVD2 and VTSIP mutations. *Biochem Biophys Res Commun.* 2002;299:594-598.
37. Beffagna G, Occhi G, Nava A, et al. Regulatory mutations in transforming growth factor-beta3 gene cause arrhythmogenic right ventricular cardiomyopathy type 1. *Cardiovasc Res.* 2005;65:366-373.
38. Merner ND, Hodgkinson KA, Haywood AF, et al. Arrhythmogenic right ventricular cardiomyopathy type 5 is a fully penetrant, lethal arrhythmic disorder caused by a missense mutation in the TMEM43 gene. *Am J Hum Genet.* 2008;82:809-821.
39. van Tintelen JP, Van Gelder IC, Asimaki A, et al. Severe cardiac phenotype with right ventricular predominance in a large cohort of patients with a single missense mutation in the DES gene. *Heart Rhythm.* 2009;6:1574-1583.
40. Otten E, Asimaki A, Maass A, et al. Desmin mutations as a cause of right ventricular heart failure affect the intercalated disks. *Heart Rhythm.* 2010;7:1058-1064.
41. Taylor M, Graw S, Sinagra G, et al. Genetic variation in titin in arrhythmogenic right ventricular cardiomyopathy-overlap syndromes. *Circulation.* 2011;124:876-885.
42. Quarta G, Syrris P, Ashworth M, et al. Mutations in the Lamin A/C gene mimic arrhythmogenic right ventricular cardiomyopathy. *Eur Heart J.* 2012;33:1128-1136.
43. van der Zwaag PA, van Rijsingen IA, Asimaki A, et al. Phospholamban R14del mutation in patients diagnosed with dilated cardiomyopathy or arrhythmogenic right ventricular cardiomyopathy: evidence supporting the concept of arrhythmogenic cardiomyopathy. *Eur J Heart Fail.* 2012;14:1199-1207.
44. Groeneweg JA, van der Zwaag PA, Jongbloed JD, et al. Left-dominant arrhythmogenic cardiomyopathy in a large family: associated desmosomal or nondesmosomal genotype? *Heart Rhythm.* 2013;10:548-559.

45. Kirchhof P, Fabritz L, Zwiener M, et al. Age- and training-dependent development of arrhythmogenic right ventricular cardiomyopathy in heterozygous plakoglobin-deficient mice. *Circulation.* 2006;114:1799-1806.
46. Fabritz L, Hoogendijk MG, Scicluna BP, et al. Load-reducing therapy prevents development of arrhythmogenic right ventricular cardiomyopathy in plakoglobin-deficient mice. *J Am Coll Cardiol.* 2011;57:740-750.
47. La Gerche A, Robberecht C, Kuiperi C, et al. Lower than expected desmosomal gene mutation prevalence in endurance athletes with complex ventricular arrhythmias of right ventricular origin. *Heart.* 2010;96:1268-1274.
48. McKenna WJ, Thiene G, Nava A, et al. Diagnosis of arrhythmogenic right ventricular dysplasia/cardiomyopathy. Task Force of the Working Group Myocardial and Pericardial Disease of the European Society of Cardiology and of the Scientific Council on Cardiomyopathies of the International Society and Federation of Cardiology. *Br Heart J.* 1994;71:215-218.
49. Marcus FI, McKenna WJ, Sherrill D, et al. Diagnosis of arrhythmogenic right ventricular cardiomyopathy/dysplasia: proposed modification of the Task Force Criteria. *Circulation.* 2010;121:1533-1541.
50. Kapplinger JD, Landstrom AP, Salisbury BA, et al. Distinguishing arrhythmogenic right ventricular cardiomyopathy/dysplasia-associated mutations from background genetic noise. *J Am Coll Cardiol.* 2011;57:2317-2327.
51. Hamid MS, Norman M, Quraishi A, et al. Prospective evaluation of relatives for familial arrhythmogenic right ventricular cardiomyopathy/dysplasia reveals a need to broaden diagnostic criteria. *J Am Coll Cardiol.* 2002; 40:1445-1450.
52. Syrris P, Ward D, Asimaki A, et al. Clincal expression of plakophilin-2 mutations in familial arrhythmogenic right ventricular cardiomyopathy. *Circulation.* 2006;113:356-364.
53. Bhuiyan ZA, Jongbloed JD, van der Smagt J, et al. Desmoglein-2 and desmocollin-2 mutations in dutch arrhythmogenic right ventricular dysplasia/cardiomypathy patients: results from a multicenter study. *Circ Cardiovasc Genet.* 2009;2:418-427.

4

Genetic Counseling for Patients and Relatives

Argelia Medeiros-Domingo, MD, PhD

Introduction

Genetic counseling is defined as the information and support provided to individuals and families at risk of genetic disease.[1] Before performing a genetic test, it is highly recommended to have a genetic counselor to properly explain the test itself and to translate the meaning and consequences of the genetic test result.

Genetic counseling sessions usually consist of a review of the patient's clinical history, family background, and a deep discussion of the genetic test results, including eventual prognostic or risk implications of the test results.[2] In ARVC/D, genetic counseling represents a great challenge. ARVC/D is most commonly transmitted as an autosomal dominant trait, with incomplete penetrance and variable phenotypic expression.[3] Affected individuals frequently have more than one genetic defect[4] in the same gene or in a second complementary gene.[5] Thus, ARVC/D genetic counseling requires a great dose of individualized medicine. Patients who have a suspected risk of ARVC/D are usually concerned about the potentially affected close relatives; the benefits of performing the test in other family members, including minors, should be also discussed. Despite having the same potential pathogenic mutation, the outcome and general scenario surrounding a particular mutation is different in each patient, even in the context of monozygotic twins;[6] thus, every case has to be evaluated in their individual contexts.

Benefits of and Indication for ARVC/D Genetic Testing

The ARVC/D genetic test, if positive, can identify patients in early stages of the disease with possible or probable phenotypes. In those with clear phenotypes, the test might provide the genetic substrate to track in other asymptomatic relatives who are potentially affected. If an ARVC/D patient wishes to conceive a

Current Concepts in Arrhythmogenic Right Ventricular Cardiomyopathy/Dysplasia

child, for example, a positive genetic test could be useful if in vitro fertilization methods are being considered, since a preimplantation genetic diagnosis could be performed.

The ARVC/D genetic test is also useful in the context of sudden cardiac death syndrome victims in whom ARVC/D is suspected. Detection of a pathogenic mutation could be of crucial value for other relatives at risk.[7]

The expert consensus statement on the state of genetic testing for channelopathies and cardiomyopathies states that in patients satisfying the 2010 Task Force Diagnostic Criteria for ARVC/D, genetic testing is indicated. They recommend considering genetic testing in patients with possible ARVC/D according to the 2010 Task Force Criteria, but do not recommended it for patients with only a single minor criterion. Mutation-specific genetic testing is also recommended for family members following the identification of the ARVC/D-causative mutation in an index case.[8] Moreover, in the 2010 Task Force Criteria, the identification of a pathogenic mutation categorized as associated or probably associated with ARVC/D is considered a major criterion in the diagnosis of the disease.[9]

What to Expect from ARVC/D Genetic Testing

Only 50% of the cases with a clear ARVC/D phenotype will have a mutation in the known genes. It is crucial to make this information clear to the patient before performing the test, so that it will be easier to explain that the absence of putative mutations does not mean absence of disease or misdiagnosis. The genetic defect could be in a genomic region not yet detected as ARVC/D-related.

It is also important to inform the patients about the characteristics of the genetic test to be performed. There are several ARVC/D genetic tests available, in research or commercial settings. These usually include the coding regions of the 5 principal desmosomal genes associated to the disease: *PKP2* (plakophilin-2), *DSG2* (desmoglein-2), *DSP* (desmoplakin), *DSC2* (desmocollin-2), and *JUP* (plakoglobin) (Figure 4.1). Less often, ARVC/D genetic tests include other novel genes like *DES* (desmin), *TTN* (titin), *TMEM43* (transmembrane protein 43), *LMNA* (lamin A/C), *PLN* (phospholamban), and *TGF-β3* (transforming growth factor-β3). If a genetic test result is "negative," the patient should have an explanation of the meaning of this negative result; the mutation might be present in a gene still not known or in a minor gene not scanned by the selected test.

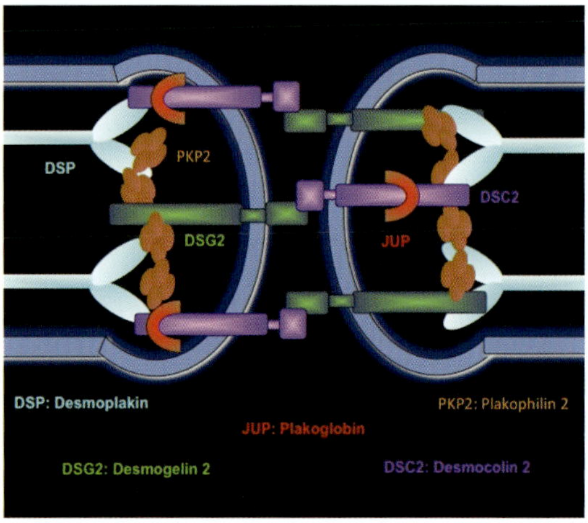

FIGURE 4.1 Desmosomal genes.

The list of ARVC/D-related genes continues to grow; nevertheless, among the 50% positives, 80% of the mutations are located in three major desmosomal genes. These are *PKP2*, *DSG2*, and *DSP* (Figure 4.2). Large DNA deletions/duplications are not commonly searched, and the precise prevalence of such mutations in ARVC/D is unknown.[10] The standard genetic test will also not detect errors in RNA transcription or processing.

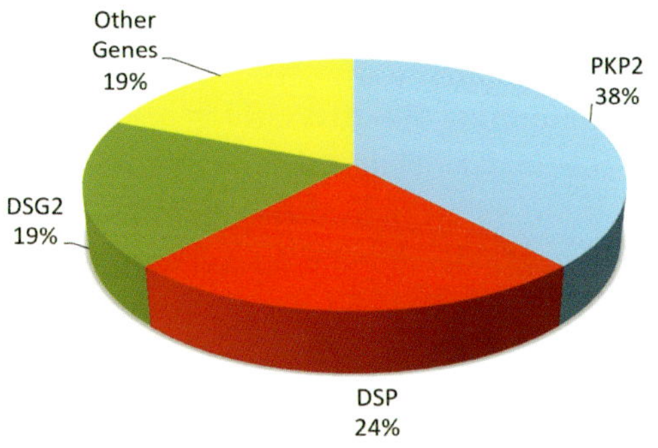

FIGURE 4.2 Distribution of mutations among the most common ARVC/D genes. Numbers are adapted from disease-associated mutations listed in the Human Gene Mutation Database as of September 2012.

The method used during the genetic test is crucial to estimate the probability of missing mutations. In the research setting, some laboratories use denaturing high-performance liquid chromatography (DHPLC) as an intermediate detection platform, which constitutes a low-cost, fast screening method with a relatively high rate of misses (up to 16%).[11] Direct Sanger sequencing has been used during the last 25 years; this method provides an excellent DNA read-out with low rate of misses (less than 2%). It is widely used, although it is expensive compared with next-generation sequencing. During the last 10 years, next-generation sequencing methods have been developing rapidly; they offer a fast sequencing methodology at low cost with a low rate of misses. Routine sequencing of large genes has been possible using this technology and is becoming the preferred method for genetic screening.

Genetic Test Interpretation

As mentioned before, genetic test interpretation should be done in an individualized manner; nevertheless, it is important to lay out some general concepts.

It has been reported that nearly 16% of the control population hosts a mutation in at least one ARVC/D gene. Usually these variants are missense mutations. Radical mutations in ARVC/D genes have a higher probability of being disease-causative; thus, rare missense mutations should be interpreted with great caution.[12] Interestingly, several studies have reported that multiple desmosomal variants are commonly seen in affected probands compared with healthy relatives.[12,13] Compound heterozygocity seems to be a common finding in ARVC/D cases (Figure 4.3).[14]

To date, more than 760 variants in the 5 major desmosomal genes have been described.[15] Less than 5% have been functionally characterized; pathogenicity is generally suspected when a variant is absent in at least 500 reference alleles and involves a conserved residue across species, and a dysfunctional protein has been predicted using several available computer simulation ("in-silico") tools like PolyPhen, an in-silico tool that predicts possible impact of amino acid substitution on the structure and function of a human protein, and SIFT, another in-silico tool that also predicts whether an amino acid substitution affects protein function based on the degree of conservation of amino acid residues

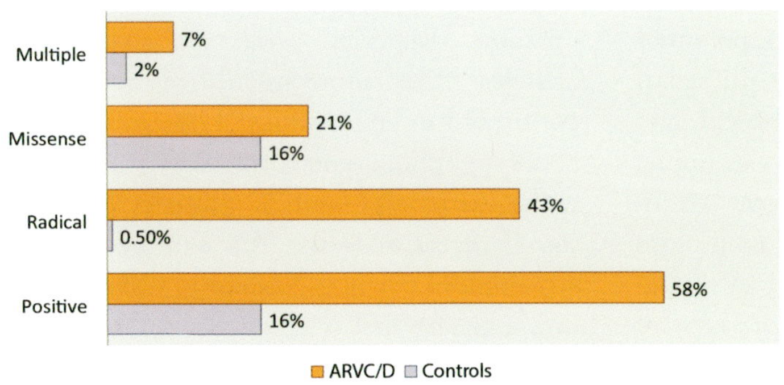

FIGURE 4.3 Characteristics of mutations found in ARVC/D cases and control population. *Source:* Adapted from Kapplinger et al.[12]

in sequence alignments derived from closely related species. Commercial and research tests have developed different classifications to assign the risk of the ARVC/D variant or variants reported. Generally speaking, variants could be classified as:

1. Pathogenic, when a variant has been proved or is predicted to be deleterious.
2. Variants of uncertain significance, when the variant is suspected to be deleterious.
3. No known pathogenicity, if a variant is not expected to cause disease.

Screening of family members is recommended when a Class I variant has been found. When a Class II variant is present, family members may benefit of genetic screening. For Class III variants, family screening is not recommended.[8]

ARVC/D is a disease with incomplete penetrance. Genetic carriers of one particular mutation might not develop the disease.[16] When a family member does not exhibit the phenotype yet carries the mutation, it is important to consider the following factors:

1. Age: the majority of cases will develop the disease after age 30.
2. Gender: males are more often affected than females. Nonetheless, gender does not have a clear effect on outcome.[17]

It is advisable to plan carefully what information should be provided to asymptomatic carriers. Before delivering any genetic test result, it is important to consider potential psychological consequences. The physician should evaluate the particular clinical scenario; the approach will differ if, for example, the physician is providing genetic counseling to a family member who lost a close relative versus to a family member of a relative with mild disease. Consider the type of mutation(s), age, and gender in order to estimate the subject's probability of developing the disease.

Performing the ARVC/D genetic test on subjects under the age of 12 is controversial,[18] because even an individual who tests positive is unlikely to develop the disease during childhood.[19,20] An ARVC/D genetic test done too early could label a child as "sick" and impair his quality of life, particularly if only variants of uncertain significance have been found in the affected relative. Nevertheless, if a radical pathogenic mutation has been detected with a high-penetrance pattern and early presentation of the disease or a recessive pattern is suspected, genetic testing might be useful to predict the risk to develop the disease and could potentially be used for prenatal counseling.

There is no early treatment proven to be useful in asymptomatic carriers; however, it has been suggested that vasodilator drugs may decrease the progression of the ventricular damage,[21] and excessive exercise appears to exacerbate the manifestation of the disease.[22] For relatives of an ARVC/D case with variants of uncertain significance or potential compound heterozygosity, clinical evaluation for ARVC/D continues to be the most important tool in disease detection[23,24] and still-imperfect risk stratification.

ARVC/D Genotype-Phenotype Correlation

To date, the ARVC/D genetic tests do not provide a clear genotype–phenotype correlation and have limited value-predicting outcome. Reported series are small; nevertheless, they show interesting data to be confirmed in larger series. The most obvious genotype–phenotype correlation in ARVC/D is the extreme phenotype given by the autosomal recessive forms, the cardiocutaneous syndromes known as Naxos and Carvajal syndromes. The first is characterized by woolly hair and palmoplantar keratoderma with early development of ARVC/D, while the second has the same skin phenotype along with left ventricular involvement, commonly with ventricular aneurysms in certain areas, and finally dilated cardiomyopathy. These phenotypes are given by homozygous mutations in plakoglobin (*JUP*) or desmoplakin (DSP).[25,26]

Fressart et al reported recently that desmosomal mutations are associated with younger age of disease presentation, multiple mutations with sudden death,[27] and *DSG2* mutations with left ventricular involvement. Patients with left ventricular involvement are known to have worse outcomes than those without.[28] Cox et al reported recently that young, asymptomatic mutation-carriers frequently exhibit prolonged terminal activation duration as a first or early sign of ARVC/D.[29] Families with *DSP* mutations have been reported to have a high occurrence of sudden death as first clinical manifestation.[30]

Many research projects are running currently with the goal of finding other prognostic applications of the ARVC/D genetic test, and in the near future, the genetic test could potentially be used for risk stratification of the disease.

References

1. Harris A, Kelly SE, Wyatt S. Counseling customers: emerging roles for genetic counselors in the direct-to-consumer genetic testing market. *J Genet Couns.* 2013;22:277-288.
2. Ingles J, Yeates L, Hunt L, et al. Health status of cardiac genetic disease patients and their at-risk relatives. *Int J Cardiol.* 2013;165:448-453.
3. Campuzano O, Alcalde M, Allegue C, et al. Genetics of arrhythmogenic right ventricular cardiomyopathy. *J Med Genet.* 2013;50:280-289.
4. Bauce B, Nava A, Beffagna G, et al. Multiple mutations in desmosomal proteins encoding genes in arrhythmogenic right ventricular cardiomyopathy/dysplasia. *Heart Rhythm.* 2010;7:22-29.
5. Marcus FI, Edson S, Towbin JA. Genetics of arrhythmogenic right ventricular cardiomyopathy: a practical guide for physicians. *J Am Coll Cardiol.* 2013;61:1945-1948.
6. Wlodarska EK, Konka M, Zaleska T, et al. Arrhythmogenic right ventricular cardiomyopathy in two pairs of monozygotic twins. *Int J Cardiol.* 2005;105:126-133.
7. Elger BS, Michaud K, Fellmann F, Mangin P. Sudden death: ethical and legal problems of post-mortem forensic genetic testing for hereditary cardiac diseases. *Clin Genet.* 2010;77:287-292.
8. Ackerman MJ, Priori SG, Willems S, et al. HRS/EHRA expert consensus statement on the state of genetic testing for the channelopathies and cardiomyopathies; this document was developed as a partnership between the Heart Rhythm Society (HRS) and the European Heart Rhythm Association (EHRA). *Heart Rhythm.* 2011;8:1308-1339.
9. Marcus FI, McKenna WJ, Sherrill D, et al. Diagnosis of arrhythmogenic right ventricular cardiomyopathy/dysplasia: proposed modification of the Task Force Criteria. *Circulation.* 2010;121:1533-1541.
10. Roberts J, Herkert J, Rutberg J, et al. Detection of genomic deletions of PKP2 in arrhythmogenic right ventricular cardiomyopathy. *Clin Genet.* 2013;83:452-456.
11. Medlock MM, Tester DJ, Will ML, Bos JM, Ackerman MJ. Repeat long QT syndrome genetic testing of phenotype-positive cases: prevalence and etiology of detection misses. *Heart Rhythm.* 2012;9:1977-1982.
12. Kapplinger JD, Landstrom AP, Salisbury BA, et al. Distinguishing arrhythmogenic right ventricular cardiomyopathy/dysplasia-associated mutations from background genetic noise. *J Am Coll Cardiol.* 2011;57:2317-2327.
13. Quarta G, Muir A, Pantazis A, et al. Familial evaluation in arrhythmogenic right ventricular cardiomyopathy: impact of genetics and revised Task Force Criteria. *Circulation.* 2011;123:2701-2709.
14. Nakajima T, Kaneko Y, Irie T, et al. Compound and digenic heterozygosity in desmosome genes as a cause of arrhythmogenic

right ventricular cardiomyopathy in Japanese patients. *Circ J*. 2012;76:737-743.
15. van der Zwaag PA, Jongbloed JD, van den Berg MP, et al. A genetic variants database for arrhythmogenic right ventricular dysplasia/cardiomyopathy. *Hum Mutat*. 2009;30: 1278-1283.
16. Aneq MA, Fluur C, Rehnberg M, et al. Novel plakophilin2 mutation: three-generation family with arrhythmogenic right ventricular cardiomyopathy. *Scand Cardiovasc J*. 2012;46: 72-75.
17. Bauce B, Frigo G, Marcus FI, et al. Comparison of clinical features of arrhythmogenic right ventricular cardiomyopathy in men versus women. *Am J Cardiol*. 2008;102:1252-1257.
18. Bauce B, Rampazzo A, Basso C, et al. Clinical phenotype and diagnosis of arrhythmogenic right ventricular cardiomyopathy in pediatric patients carrying desmosomal gene mutations. *Heart Rhythm*. 2011;8:1686-1695.
19. Ohno S, Nagaoka I, Fukuyama M, et al. Age-dependent clinical and genetic characteristics in Japanese patients with arrhythmogenic right ventricular cardiomyopathy/dysplasia. *Circ J*. 2013;77(6):1534-1542.
20. Corrado D, Basso C, Thiene G, et al. Spectrum of clinicopathologic manifestations of arrhythmogenic right ventricular cardiomyopathy/dysplasia: a multicenter study. *J Am Coll Cardiol*. 1997;30:1512-1520.
21. Fabritz L, Fortmuller L, Yu TY, Paul M, Kirchhof P. Can preload-reducing therapy prevent disease progression in arrhythmogenic right ventricular cardiomyopathy? Experimental evidence and concept for a clinical trial. *Prog Biophys Mol Biol*. 2012;110:340-346.
22. Heidbuchel H, La Gerche A. The right heart in athletes. Evidence for exercise-induced arrhythmogenic right ventricular cardiomyopathy. *Herzschrittmacherther Elektrophysiol*. 2012;23:82-86.
23. Marcus FI, Abidov A. Arrhythmogenic right ventricular cardiomyopathy 2012: diagnostic challenges and treatment. *J Cardiovasc Electrophysiol*. 2012;23:1149-1153.
24. Smith W. Guidelines for the diagnosis and management of arrhythmogenic right ventricular cardiomyopathy. *Heart Lung Circ*. 2011;20:757-760.
25. Alcalai R, Metzger S, Rosenheck S, Meiner V, Chajek-Shaul T. A recessive mutation in desmoplakin causes arrhythmogenic right ventricular dysplasia, skin disorder, and woolly hair. *J Am Coll Cardiol*. 2003;42:319-327.
26. Protonotarios N, Tsatsopoulou A. Naxos disease and Carvajal syndrome: cardiocutaneous disorders that highlight the pathogenesis and broaden the spectrum of arrhythmogenic right ventricular cardiomyopathy. *Cardiovasc Pathol*. 2004;13:185-194.
27. Fressart V, Duthoit G, Donal E, et al. Desmosomal gene analysis in arrhythmogenic right ventricular dysplasia/cardiomyopathy: spectrum of mutations and clinical impact in practice. *Europace*. 2010;12:861-868.
28. Pinamonti B, Dragos AM, Pyxaras SA, et al. Prognostic predictors in arrhythmogenic right ventricular cardiomyopathy: results from a 10-year registry. *Eur Heart J*. 2011;32: 1105-1113.
29. Cox MG, van der Zwaag PA, van der Werf C, et al. Arrhythmogenic right ventricular dysplasia/cardiomyopathy: pathogenic desmosome mutations in index-patients predict outcome of family screening: Dutch arrhythmogenic right ventricular dysplasia/cardiomyopathy genotype–phenotype follow-up study. *Circulation*. 2011;123:2690-2700.
30. Bauce B, Basso C, Rampazzo A, et al. Clinical profile of four families with arrhythmogenic right ventricular cardiomyopathy caused by dominant desmoplakin mutations. *Eur Heart J*. 2005;26:1666-1675.

5

Arrhythmogenic Right Ventricular Cardiomyopathy/Dysplasia: Clinical Presentation, Differential Diagnosis, and Diagnostic Challenges

Rajesh Janardhanan, MD, and Frank I. Marcus, MD

Clinical Presentation

Arrhythmogenic right ventricular cardiomyopathy/dysplasia (ARVC/D) is a genetically determined heart muscle disorder that is characterized pathologically by fibrofatty replacement of the right ventricular (RV) myocardium. There is a predilection for the male sex with onset of clinical symptoms mostly in the second to fourth decades of life.[1] ARVC/D is present in approximately 5% of individuals who experience sudden cardiac death (SCD) and may be more common among athletes who die suddenly.[2] The clinical diagnosis of ARVC/D is complex, since there is no single diagnostic "gold standard"; diagnosis is based on major and minor criteria that have been modified and take into account heart structure and function, family history, genetic mutations, histology, ventricular arrhythmias, and electrocardiographic (ECG) abnormalities (Table 5.1).[3]

The most typical clinical presentation consists of palpitations or syncope. Cardiac arrest or SCD may also be the initial presentation. Ventricular tachycardia (VT) of left bundle branch block (LBBB) morphology should raise the possibility of ARVC/D. The presence of T-wave inversions in leads V_1–V_3 or beyond on a routine 12-lead ECG may be the initial finding in an otherwise normal individual. Other typical presentations may include frequent premature ventricular contractions (PVCs) of LBBB morphology or nonsustained VT. There usually are RV abnormalities such as enlargement, wall motion abnormalities, decreased function, and/or localized aneurysms (Figure 5.1).

Disease expression is variable. ECG changes and arrhythmias may develop before histologic evidence of myocyte loss or clinical evidence of RV dysfunction.[4] Clinical manifestations vary with age and disease stage.[5] In the early "concealed phase," individuals are

TABLE 5.1 ARVC/D Revised Task Force Criteria[3]

I. GLOBAL OR REGIONAL DYSFUNCTION AND STRUCTURAL ALTERATIONS	
MAJOR	**By 2D echocardiography:** Regional RV akinesia, dyskinesia, or aneurysm **and** 1 of the following (end diastole): • PLAX RVOT ≥ 32 mm (corrected for body size [PLAX/BSA] ≥ 19 mm/m^2) • PSAX RVOT ≥ 36 mm (corrected for body size [PSAX/BSA] ≥ 21 mm/m^2) • **or** fractional area change ≤ 33%
MAJOR	**By MRI:** Regional RV akinesia or dyskinesia or dyssynchronous RV contraction **and** one of the following: • Ratio of RV end-diastolic volume to BSA ≥ 110 mL/m^2 (male) or ≥ 100 mL/m^2 (female) • **or** RV ejection fraction ≤ 40%
MAJOR	**By RV angiography:** Regional RV akinesia, dyskinesia, or aneurysm
MINOR	**By 2D echocardiography:*** Regional RV akinesia or dyskinesia **and** one of the following (end diastole): • PLAX RVOT ≥ 29 to < 32 mm (corrected for body size [PLAX/BSA] ≥ 16 to < 19 mm/m^2) • PSAX RVOT ≥ 32 to < 36 mm (corrected for body size [PSAX/BSA] ≥ 18 to < 21 mm/m^2) • **or** fractional area change > 33% to ≤ 40%
MINOR	**By MRI:*** Regional RV akinesia or dyskinesia or dyssynchronous RV contraction and one of the following: • Ratio of RV end-diastolic volume to BSA ≥ 100 to < 110 mL/m^2 (male) • **or** ≥ 90 to < 100 mL/m^2 (female) • **or** RV ejection fraction > 40% to ≤ 45%
	II. TISSUE CHARACTERIZATION OF WALL
MAJOR	Residual myocytes < 60% by morphometric analysis (or < 50% if estimated), with fibrous replacement of the RV free wall myocardium in ≥ 1 sample, with or without fatty replacement of tissue on endomyocardial biopsy
MINOR	Residual myocytes 60% to 75% by morphometric analysis (or 50% to 65% if estimated), with fibrous replacement of the RV free wall myocardium in ≥ 1 sample, with or without fatty replacement of tissue on endomyocardial biopsy
	III. REPOLARIZATION ABNORMALITIES
MAJOR	Inverted T waves in right precordial leads (V_1, V_2, and V_3) or beyond in individuals > 14 years of age (in the absence of complete right bundle branch block QRS ≥ 120 ms)
MINOR	Inverted T waves in leads V_1 and V_2 in individuals > 14 years of age (in the absence of complete right bundle branch block) or in V_4, V_5, or V_6
	Inverted T waves in leads V_1, V_2, V_3, and V_4 in individuals > 14 years of age in the presence of complete right bundle branch block
	IV. DEPOLARIZATION/CONDUCTION ABNORMALITIES
MAJOR	Epsilon wave (reproducible low-amplitude signals between end of QRS complex to onset of the T wave) in the right precordial leads (V_1 to V_3)
MINOR	Late potentials by SAECG in ≥ 1 of 3 parameters in the absence of a QRS duration of ≥ 110 ms on the standard ECG
	Filtered QRS duration (fQRS) ≥ 114 ms
	Duration of terminal QRS < 40 µV (low-amplitude signal duration) ≥ 38 ms
	Root-mean-square voltage of terminal 40 ms ≤ 20 µV
	Terminal activation duration of QRS ≥ 55 ms measured from the nadir of the S wave to the end of the QRS, including R', in V_1, V_2, or V_3, in the absence of complete right bundle branch block

	V. ARRHYTHMIAS
MAJOR	Nonsustained or sustained ventricular tachycardia of left bundle branch morphology with superior axis (negative or indeterminate QRS in leads II, III, and aVF and positive in lead aVL)
MINOR	Nonsustained or sustained ventricular tachycardia of RV outflow configuration, left bundle branch block morphology with inferior axis (positive QRS in leads II, III, and aVF and negative in lead aVL) or of unknown axis > 500 ventricular extrasystoles per 24 hours (Holter)
	VI. FAMILY HISTORY
MAJOR	ARVC/D confirmed in a first-degree relative who meets current Task Force Criteria
	ARVC/D confirmed pathologically at autopsy or surgery in a first-degree relative
	† Identification of a pathogenic mutation categorized as associated or probably associated with ARVC/D in the patient under evaluation
MINOR	History of ARVC/D in a first-degree relative in whom it is not possible or practical to determine whether the family member meets current Task Force Criteria
	Premature sudden death (< 35 years of age) due to suspected ARVC/D in a first-degree relative
	ARVC/D confirmed pathologically or by current Task Force Criteria in second-degree relative

PLAX indicates parasternal long-axis view; RVOT, RV outflow tract; BSA, body surface area; PSAX, parasternal short-axis view; aVF, augmented voltage unipolar left foot lead; and aVL, augmented voltage unipolar left arm lead.

*Hypokinesis is not included in this or subsequent definitions of RV regional wall motion abnormalities for the modified criteria.

†A pathogenic mutation is a DNA alteration associated with ARVC/D that alters or is expected to alter the encoded protein, is unobserved or rare in a large non-ARVC/D control population, and either alters or is predicted to alter the structure or function of the protein or has demonstrated linkage to the disease phenotype in a conclusive pedigree.

Diagnostic terminology for revised criteria: DEFINITE DIAGNOSIS: 2 major or 1 major and 2 minor criteria or 4 minor from different categories; BORDERLINE: 1 major and 1 minor or 3 minor criteria from different categories; POSSIBLE: 1 major or 2 minor criteria from different categories.

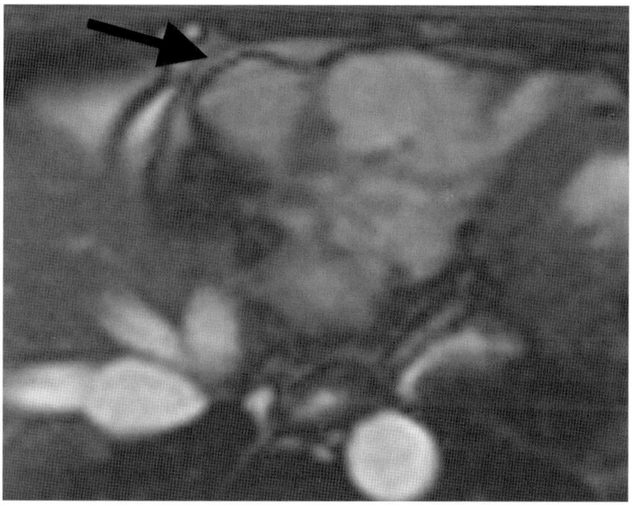

FIGURE 5.1 Axial slice of the right ventricle on cardiac MRI from a patient with ARVC/D. (**Black arrow** points to areas of regional dyskinesia and aneurysm formation on the RV free wall.)

often asymptomatic but may nonetheless be at risk for SCD, particularly during exertion.[2] In the overt "electrical phase," individuals present with symptomatic arrhythmias, and RV morphologic abnormalities are readily discernible by conventional imaging. Later, diffuse disease may result in RV or biventricular heart failure. The ultimate phenotype may resemble dilated cardiomyopathy (end-stage disease). In the past, left ventricular (LV) involvement was considered an expression of the advanced disease phase. However, the disease can start with isolated or predominant LV involvement in the early stages, even in the absence of systolic dysfunction.[6]

Diagnosis of Familial ARVC/D

In the setting of a positive family history, even minor ECG and echocardiographic abnormalities are important and often diagnostic (Table 5.2).[7,8] Details of the genetic abnormalities and their implications are addressed in another chapter.

Differential Diagnosis

The diagnosis of ARVC/D relies on the demonstration of structural, functional, and electrophysiologic abnormalities that are caused by the underlying histologic changes. The diagnosis can be challenging in the early stage ("concealed phase") in the absence of overt structural changes.

In endurance athletes, training can lead to RV enlargement, ECG abnormalities, and arrhythmias, reflecting the increased hemodynamic load during exercise.[9] Global RV systolic dysfunction or regional wall motion abnormalities can indicate ARVC/D rather than physiologic ventricular enlargement.

The pathologic diagnosis of ARVC/D is based on histologic demonstration of fibrofatty replacement of RV myocardium on biopsy, necropsy, or surgery.[10] RV endomyocardial biopsy has limited sensitivity because the segmental nature of the disease may cause false-negative results. Use of electroanatomic voltage mapping to identify pathologic areas for biopsy sampling may improve the yield.[11] The recognition of myocyte loss with fibrous or fibrofatty replacement can be valuable diagnostically. RV free wall biopsy carries a slight risk of perforation, but the more accessible interventricular septum rarely exhibits histologic changes.[12] Nevertheless, septal biopsy may identify other conditions such as sarcoidosis, myocarditis, and endomyocardial fibrosis.

The differential diagnosis of ARVC/D includes idiopathic RV outflow tachycardia, sarcoidosis, myocarditis, dilated cardiomyopathy, Chagas disease, RV infarction, and Brugada syndrome. Congenital heart disease with right chamber overload, such as Ebstein

TABLE 5.2 Diagnosis of ARVC/D in a family member[7]

In the context of ARVC/D in a first-degree relative, the diagnosis of familial ARVC/D is based on the documentation of ONE of the following in a family member:	
ECG	T-wave inversion in right precordial leads V_1, V_2, and V_3 in individuals > 14 years
SAECG	Presence of late potentials on SAECG
Arrhythmias	Ventricular tachycardia of LBBB morphology on ECG, Holter monitor, or during exercise testing or > 200 PVCs in 24 hours
Structural or functional abnormalities of the RV	Either mild global dilatation or reduction in RV ejection fraction with normal LV or mild segmental dilatation of the RV or regional RV hypokinesis

PVC = premature ventricular contractions; SAECG = signal-averaged ECG anomaly, atrial septal defect, Uhl anomaly, and pulmonary hypertension, are other clinical phenocopies.[1] Catecholaminergic polymorphic ventricular tachycardia is considered a disorder distinct from ARVC/D.[13]

Idiopathic RV outflow tachycardia, a benign nonfamilial condition, is an important and challenging differential diagnosis. The absence of ECG repolarization/depolarization abnormalities and RV structural changes, as well as the recording of a single VT morphology and noninducibility at programmed ventricular stimulation with a normal voltage map, provides evidence for the idiopathic nature of the VT.[14] A scoring system[15] that can distinguish RV outflow tract tachycardia in patients with ARVC/D from that in patients with idiopathic VT consists of the following: During sinus rhythm in patients with ARVC/D, there may be T-wave inversions in leads V_1–V_3. During VT in patients with ARVC/D, the QRS duration in lead 1 is ≥ 120 ms. There is QRS notching and the precordial transition is present in lead V_5 or later.

Myocardial involvement in sarcoidosis can mimic the clinical and structural abnormalities of ARVC/D.[16] In a prospective study of consecutive patients with suspected ARVC/D evaluated by a standard protocol including biopsy, a surprisingly high incidence (15%) of cardiac sarcoid was found.[17] The similarity in clinical presentation and cardiovascular magnetic resonance imaging (MRI) findings can pose a challenge in differentiating between the 2 conditions in the absence of histologic diagnosis. The current diagnostic ARVC/D guidelines do not reliably exclude patients with cardiac sarcoidosis. Clinical and electrophysiologic parameters in cardiac sarcoid that may help include reduced LV ejection fraction, a significantly wider QRS complex, right-sided apical VT, and more inducible forms of monomorphic VT.[18]

It has been suggested that patients with ARVC/D may be susceptible to viral myocarditis, which could lead to a decrease in cardiac function and accelerate disease progression.[19] The presence of a pathologic mutation and the addition of myocarditis or volume loading may trigger overt manifestations of ARVC/D, a phenomenon that has been seen in some animal models.[20] The link between ARVC/D and myocarditis is still undefined.

Diagnostic Challenges

Electrocardiography. Inverted T waves in right precordial leads (V_1–V_3) may be a normal finding in children under 14 years of age. It may also be present in less than 1% of older normal individuals.[21] In individuals over 14 years of age (in the absence of complete RBBB with QRS complex duration ≥ 120 ms), the presence of inverted T waves in right precordial leads (V_1–V_3 or beyond) is a major criterion in the revised Task Force Criteria.[3] Its prevalence in ARVC/D has been reported as 55% to 94% in different series.[22] The extent of right precordial T-wave inversion relates to the degree of RV involvement.

Arrhythmias of RV origin with LBBB morphology is a cardinal feature of ARVC/D but can occur in other diseases, particularly in idiopathic RV outflow tract tachycardia.

The presence of LBBB VT with an inferior axis (R-wave positive in leads II and III and negative in lead aVL) is typical of focal RV outflow tract tachycardia.[23] Similar features may be seen in patients with ARVC/D but usually coexist with anterior T-wave inversion and ventricular arrhythmias of varying morphologies.

Depolarization delay in right precordial leads is also common in ARVC/D. Evaluation of the duration of terminal QRS complex activation incorporates slurring of the S wave, as well as the R', into a single measure of terminal activation duration.[24] However, T-wave inversion in leads V_1, V_2, and

V_3 extending to V_4 is uncommon in patients with RBBB who do not have ARVC/D and is seen frequently in those who do have the disease.

Imaging. Technical advances in cardiac MRI and echocardiography have improved the ability to image the RV with reproducible measurements of volume and systolic function, and permit classification of severity and differentiation from normals.[25] Cardiac MRI is commonly used in patients with suspected ARVC/D. Previous diagnostic reliance on subjective assessment of RV wall thinning, wall motion abnormalities, and fatty infiltration of the myocardium by CMR are probably not reliable.[26,27]

During the initial experiences with cardiac MRI in ARVC/D, the focus was on the ability of MRI to detect fatty tissue in the RV free wall. It soon became evident that this finding is of limited diagnostic specificity in the absence of concomitant wall motion abnormalities. In addition, there was also a high degree of interobserver variability.[26] The amount of subepicardial fat increases with body weight and age.[28] The presence of extensive fatty infiltration of the RV has not been found to be familial and is not associated with arrhythmic death during exercise.[29] Therefore, recognition of significant fatty involvement without concomitant fibrosis of the RV in normal individuals renders this unique capability of MRI to be of limited value. Incorrect interpretation of the MRI study is often a frequent cause of misdiagnosis of ARVC/D.[27] To a large extent, this has been mitigated with the revised Task Force Criteria,[3] which includes specific imaging guidelines.

Late gadolinium enhancement on cardiac MRI permits myocardial tissue characterization in the LV. It can be difficult to be certain of late gadolinium enhancement for characterization of RV myocardium because of the thin wall of the RV and possible confusion with fat.[30]

Pathologies causing RV volume overload such as intracardiac shunts (eg, atrial septal defects, anomalous pulmonary venous drainage) can be misinterpreted as possible ARVC/D on standard echocardiography.[31] A clue to the correct diagnosis may be the presence of a dilated RV with normal or supernormal function and without regional wall motion abnormalities in these other conditions.

Cardiac MRI can define the diagnostic features of ARVC/D, but it may also detect other diseases that can mimic ARVC/D. Quarta et al[31] analyzed 657 CMR referrals suspicious for ARVC/D in a single tertiary referral center. Potential ARVC/D mimics were grouped into 3 categories: (1) displacement of the heart, (2) RV overload, and (3) ARVC/D-like cardiac scarring. For each, a judgment of clinical impact was made. They found 20 patients (3.0%) who fulfilled imaging criteria for a diagnosis of ARVC/D. Thirty other patients (4.6%) had a potential ARVC/D mimic, of which 25 (3.8%) were considered clinically important. These results have important consequences for both patients and their families. Clinical assessment of the patients is, therefore, critical in the diagnosis of ARVC/D in addition to the detection of major and minor imaging criteria.

Genetic Testing. Individuals who have the familial genetic defect may not have any clinical manifestations and may have a normal life expectancy without developing the disease. Thus the genetic–phenotypic relationship is quite variable.[32] It must be noted that 5% to 20% of patients with the diagnosis of ARVC/D may have 2 genetic abnormalities located either on the same protein, such as plakophilin, or on another desmosomal protein (compound and digenic heterozygosity).[33] Individuals with 2 desmosomal genetic defects have a greater chance of having phenotypic expression of the disease and are often more severely affected.[34] Interpretation of genetic abnormalities is complicated by the fact that up to 16% of normal controls may have a desmosomal genetic abnormality. Therefore, a genetic abnormality must be interpreted with great caution, and genetic counseling is recommended.[32]

Conclusion

The accurate diagnosis of ARVC/D is critically important because the diagnosis carries a risk of sudden cardiac death. An incorrect diagnosis can lead to unnecessary insertion of an implantable cardioverter-defibrillator, elevate the patient's psychosocial burden, and initiate costly and extensive screening of family members, with the possibility of overdiagnosis due to inaccurate interpretation of tests performed during screening.[35] The modifications[3] of the original Task Force Criteria represent a framework to improve the diagnosis and management of ARVC/D. The revised Task Force Criteria have increased diagnostic sensitivity, particularly in dominant ARVC/D.[36]

Abbreviations

LBBB	left bundle branch block
LV	left ventricle, left ventricular
MRI	magnetic resonance imaging
PVC	premature ventricular contraction
RBBB	right bundle branch block
SCD	sudden cardiac death
VF	ventricular fibrillation
VT	ventricular tachycardia

References

1. Basso C, Corrado D, Marcus FI, Nava A, Thiene G. Arrhythmogenic right ventricular cardiomyopathy. *Lancet*. 2009;373:1289-1300.
2. Thiene G, Nava A, Corrado D, Rossi L, Pennelli N. Right ventricular cardiomyopathy and sudden death in young people. *N Engl J Med*. 1988;318:129-133.
3. Marcus FI, McKenna WJ, Sherrill D, et al. Diagnosis of arrhythmogenic right ventricular cardiomyopathy/dysplasia: proposed modification of the Task Force Criteria. *Circulation*. 2010;121:1533-1541.
4. Kaplan SR, Gard JJ, Protonotarios N, et al. Remodeling of myocyte gap junctions in arrhythmogenic right ventricular cardiomyopathy due to a deletion in plakoglobin (Naxos disease). *Heart Rhythm*. 2004;1:3-11.
5. Sen-Chowdhry S, Syrris P, Ward D, Asimaki A, Sevdalis E, McKenna WJ. Clinical and genetic characterization of families with arrhythmogenic right ventricular dysplasia/cardiomyopathy provides novel insights into patterns of disease expression. *Circulation*. 2007;115:1710-1720.
6. Basso C, Corrado D, Bauce B, Thiene G. Arrhythmogenic right ventricular cardiomyopathy. *Circ Arrhythm Electrophysiol*. 2012;5:1233-1246.
7. Hamid MS, Norman M, Quraishi A, et al. Prospective evaluation of relatives for familial arrhythmogenic right ventricular cardiomyopathy/dysplasia reveals a need to broaden diagnostic criteria. *J Am Coll Cardiol*. 2002;40:1445-1450.
8. Nava A, Bauce B, Basso C, et al. Clinical profile and long-term follow-up of 37 families with arrhythmogenic right ventricular cardiomyopathy. *J Am Coll Cardiol*. 2000;36:2226-2233.
9. Bauce B, Frigo G, Benini G, et al. Differences and similarities between arrhythmogenic right ventricular cardiomyopathy and athlete's heart adaptations. *Br J Sports Med*. 2010;44:148-154.
10. Basso C, Burke M, Fornes P, et al. Guidelines for autopsy investigation of sudden cardiac death. *Virchows Arch*. 2008;452:11-18.
11. Avella A, d'Amati G, Pappalardo A, et al. Diagnostic value of endomyocardial biopsy guided by electroanatomic voltage mapping in arrhythmogenic right ventricular cardiomyopathy/dysplasia. *J Cardiovasc Electrophysiol*. 2008;19:1127-1134.
12. Basso C, Ronco F, Marcus F, et al. Quantitative assessment of endomyocardial biopsy

in arrhythmogenic right ventricular cardiomyopathy/dysplasia: an in vitro validation of diagnostic criteria. *Eur Heart J*. 2008;29:2760-2771.

13. Awad MM, Calkins H, Judge DP. Mechanisms of disease: molecular genetics of arrhythmogenic right ventricular dysplasia/cardiomyopathy. *Nat Clin Pract Cardiovasc Med*. 2008;5:258-267.
14. Corrado D, Basso C, Leoni L, et al. Three-dimensional electroanatomical voltage mapping and histologic evaluation of myocardial substrate in right ventricular outflow tract tachycardia. *J Am Coll Cardiol*. 2008;51:731-739.
15. Hoffmayer KS, Bhave PD, Marcus GM, et al. An electrocardiographic scoring system for distinguishing right ventricular outflow tract arrhythmias in patients with arrhythmogenic right ventricular cardiomyopathy from idiopathic ventricular tachycardia. *Heart Rhythm*. 2013;10:477-482.
16. Yared K, Johri AM, Soni AV, et al. Cardiac sarcoidosis imitating arrhythmogenic right ventricular dysplasia. *Circulation*. 2008;118:e113-115.
17. Vasaiwala SC, Finn C, Delpriore J, et al. Prospective study of cardiac sarcoid mimicking arrhythmogenic right ventricular dysplasia. *J Cardiovasc Electrophysiol*. 2009;20:473-476.
18. Dechering DG, Kochhauser S, Wasmer K, et al. Electrophysiological characteristics of ventricular tachyarrhythmias in cardiac sarcoidosis versus arrhythmogenic right ventricular cardiomyopathy. *Heart Rhythm*. 2013;10:158-164.
19. Basso C, Thiene G, Corrado D, Angelini A, Nava A, Valente M. Arrhythmogenic right ventricular cardiomyopathy. Dysplasia, dystrophy, or myocarditis? *Circulation*. 1996;94: 983-991.
20. Kirchhof P, Fabritz L, Zwiener M, et al. Age- and training-dependent development of arrhythmogenic right ventricular cardiomyopathy in heterozygous plakoglobin-deficient mice. *Circulation*. 2006;114:1799-1806.
21. Nava A, Canciani B, Buja G, et al. Electrovectorcardiographic study of negative T waves on precordial leads in arrhythmogenic right ventricular dysplasia: relationship with right ventricular volumes. *J Electrocardiol*. 1988;21:239-245.
22. Peters S, Trummel M. Diagnosis of arrhythmogenic right ventricular dysplasia-cardiomyopathy: value of standard ECG revisited. *Ann Noninvasive Electrocardiol*. 2003;8:238-245.
23. Ainsworth CD, Skanes AC, Klein GJ, Gula LJ, Yee R, Krahn AD. Differentiating arrhythmogenic right ventricular cardiomyopathy from right ventricular outflow tract ventricular tachycardia using multilead QRS duration and axis. *Heart Rhythm*. 2006;3:416-423.
24. Cox MG, Nelen MR, Wilde AA, et al. Activation delay and VT parameters in arrhythmogenic right ventricular dysplasia/cardiomyopathy: toward improvement of diagnostic ECG criteria. *J Cardiovasc Electrophysiol*. 2008;19:775-781.
25. Tandri H, Daya SK, Nasir K, et al. Normal reference values for the adult right ventricle by magnetic resonance imaging. *Am J Cardiol*. 2006;98:1660-1664.
26. Bluemke DA, Krupinski EA, Ovitt T, et al. MR imaging of arrhythmogenic right ventricular cardiomyopathy: morphologic findings and interobserver reliability. *Cardiology*. 2003;99:153-162.
27. Bomma C, Rutberg J, Tandri H, et al. Misdiagnosis of arrhythmogenic right ventricular dysplasia/cardiomyopathy. *J Cardiovasc Electrophysiol*. 2004;15:300-306.
28. Shirani J, Berezowski K, Roberts WC. Quantitative measurement of normal and excessive (cor adiposum) subepicardial adipose tissue, its clinical significance, and its effect on electrocardiographic QRS voltage. *Am J Cardiol*. 1995;76:414-418.
29. Burke AP, Farb A, Tashko G, Virmani R. Arrhythmogenic right ventricular cardiomyopathy and fatty replacement of the right ventricular myocardium: are they different diseases? *Circulation*. 1998;97:1571-1580.
30. Tandri H, Saranathan M, Rodriguez ER, et al. Noninvasive detection of myocardial fibrosis in arrhythmogenic right ventricular cardiomyopathy using delayed-enhancement mag-

netic resonance imaging. *J Am Coll Cardiol.* 2005;45:98-103.

31. Quarta G, Husain SI, Flett AS, et al. Arrhythmogenic right ventricular cardiomyopathy mimics: role of cardiovascular magnetic resonance. *J Cardiovasc Magn Reson.* 2013;15:16.
32. Marcus FI, Abidov A. Arrhythmogenic right ventricular cardiomyopathy 2012: diagnostic challenges and treatment. *J Cardiovasc Electrophysiol.* 2012;23:1149-1153.
33. Xu T, Yang Z, Vatta M, et al. Multidisciplinary Study of Right Ventricular Dysplasia I. Compound and digenic heterozygosity contributes to arrhythmogenic right ventricular cardiomyopathy. *J Am Coll Cardiol.* 2010;55:587-597.
34. Quarta G, Muir A, Pantazis A, et al. Familial evaluation in arrhythmogenic right ventricular cardiomyopathy: impact of genetics and revised Task Force Criteria. *Circulation.* 2011;123:2701-2709.
35. Marcus F, Basso C, Gear K, Sorrell VL. Pitfalls in the diagnosis of arrhythmogenic right ventricular cardiomyopathy/dysplasia. *Am J Cardiol.* 2010;105:1036-1039.
36. Protonotarios N, Anastasakis A, Antoniades L, et al. Arrhythmogenic right ventricular cardiomyopathy/dysplasia on the basis of the revised diagnostic criteria in affected families with desmosomal mutations. *Eur Heart J.* 2011;32:1097-1104.

6A

The Role of Echocardiography in Arrhythmogenic Right Ventricular Cardiomyopathy/Dysplasia

Alessandra Vecchiati, MD, and Felix C. Tanner, MD

Introduction

Arrhythmogenic right ventricular cardiomyopathy/dysplasia (ARVC/D) is a genetically determined myocardial disease that predominantly affects the right ventricle (RV). It is characterized by progressive fibrofatty replacement and thinning of the RV myocardium.[1] In the early stages, these alterations may be subtle; however, they are progressive and usually involve the so-called triangle of dysplasia, affecting the inflow tract, the outflow tract, and the apex of the RV. In the late stages, diffuse RV disease and left ventricular (LV) involvement, typically evident in the posterior and lateral wall, may occur.[2] Finally, ventricular failure and ventricular arrhythmias develop as a consequence of these degenerative alterations.

Role of Echocardiography in Diagnosis of ARVC/D

The diagnostic criteria developed by the ARVC/D Task Force are based on structural, histological, electrocardiographic, arrhythmic, and genetic features of the disease.[3] Originally, the criteria were very specific, but not sensitive enough to allow detection in the early stages of the disease; therefore, they were modified recently.[4]

Possible abnormalities are divided into major and minor categories according to the specificity of their association with ARVC/D.[4] The presence of 2 major criteria, 1 major and 2 minor criteria, or 4 minor criteria from different diagnostic categories allows a definite diagnosis of ARVC/D. In contrast, a borderline diagnosis of ARVC/D is made if 1 major and 1 minor or, alternatively, 3 minor criteria from different categories are present. In addition, a possible diagnosis of ARVC/D can be considered in the presence of 1 major or 2 minor criteria from different diagnostic categories.

The features of ARVC/D as assessed by imaging are determined by the underlying structural alterations. Degeneration of cardio-

 Cardiotext Publishing, ISBN: 978-1-935395-92-8

myocytes and their replacement by fibrofatty tissue induces (1) wall motion abnormalities such as akinesia or dyskinesia, (2) wall thinning and formation of aneurysms, and (3) ventricular dilatation and reduced ejection fraction (Figure 6A.1). Such features are first detected as focal changes, at later stages typically in the triangle of dysplasia, and finally in a diffuse manner.[5-7] Echocardiography has been a valuable tool for detection of these changes for decades.[8-10]

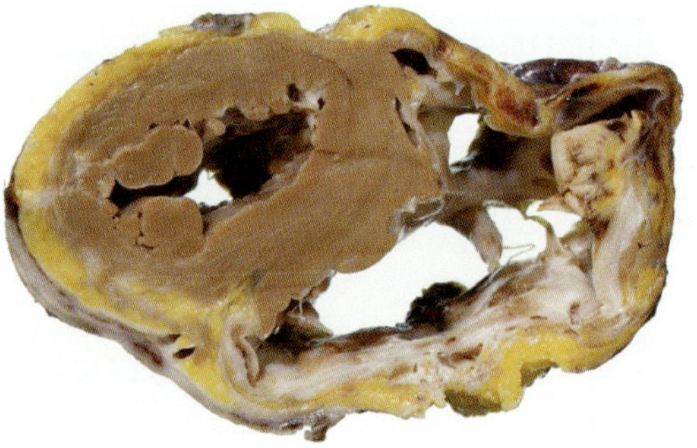

FIGURE 6A.1 Pathology specimen of a human heart affected by ARVC/D. Focal areas with degeneration of cardiac myocytes lead to replacement of the myocardium by fibrofatty tissue. These changes progress from an initially epicardial to finally transmural involvement. As a result, progressive thinning of the RV wall with aneurysm formation and ventricular dilatation occurs. The affected myocardial areas show wall motion abnormalities with hypokinesia, akinesia, or dyskinesia depending on the severity of myocardial involvement.

The structural alterations induced by ARVC/D constitute the basis for 1 major and 1 minor imaging criteria in the modified Task Force Criteria.[4] These imaging criteria are based on global or regional ventricular dysfunction as well as structural alterations, and are applied for different imaging modalities (echocardiography, cardiac magnetic resonance imaging, or RV angiography). The extent of the functional impairment or structural alterations determines whether a major or a minor criterion is fulfilled in a given patient (Table 6A.1). A major echocardiographic criterion is fulfilled with regional RV akinesia, dyskinesia, or aneurysm and one of the following: parasternal long axis (PLAX) RV outflow tract (RVOT) $\geq$ 32 mm (corrected for body size [PLAX/BSA] $\geq$ 19 mm/m^2), or parasternal short axis RVOT (PSAX) $\geq$ 36 mm (corrected for body size [PSAX/BSA] $\geq$ 21 mm/m^2), or fractional area change $\leq$ 33%. A minor echocardiographic criterion is fulfilled with regional right ventricular akinesia or dyskinesia and PLAX RVOT from $\geq$ 29 mm to < 32 mm (corrected for body size [PLAX/BSA] $\geq$ 16 mm/m^2 to < 19 mm/m^2) or PSAX RVOT from $\geq$ 32 mm to < 36 mm (corrected for body size [PSAX/BSA] $\geq$ 18 mm/m^2 to < 21 mm/m^2), or fractional area change from > 33% to $\leq$ 40%.[4]

Echocardiographic Assessment of the Right Ventricle in ARVC/D

Right Ventricular Anatomy

Although the Task Force Criteria are clearly defined, evaluation of RV size and function by standard 2D transthoracic echocardiography is difficult due to the complex geometry of the right ventricle. In contrast to the symmetrical and almost conical shape of the LV, the RV is more triangular in shape, curves over the LV, and appears like a crescent on cross-section. It is composed of 3 distinct portions—the inflow tract, the apical trabeculated part, and the outflow tract—and its blood supply is mainly provided by the right coronary artery.[11,12] Because of this complex shape, quantification of RV volume and function is challenging, as many assumptions are required. Hence, the accurate assessment of RV morphology and function requires integration of multiple echocardiographic views, including parasternal long axis, parasternal short axis, apical 4-chamber, and subcostal views (Figures 6A.2–6A.4).[13] Although different methods for quantitative echocardiographic assessment of the RV have

TABLE 6A.1 The role of echocardiography in the revised Task Force Criteria for ARVC/D

	ORIGINAL TASK FORCE CRITERIA	REVISED TASK FORCE CRITERIA
Global or regional dysfunction and structural alterations*		
MAJOR	• Severe dilation and reduction of RV ejection fraction with no (or only mild) LV impairment • Localized RV aneurysms (akinetic or dyskinetic areas with diastolic bulging) • Severe segmental dilation of the RV	**By 2D echo:** • Regional RV akinesia, dyskinesia, or aneurysm • *and* one of the following (end diastole): – PLAX RVOT ≥ 32 mm (corrected for body size [PLAX/BSA] ≥ 29 mm/m^2) – PSAX RVOT ≥ 36 mm (corrected for body size [PSAX/BSA] ≥ 29 mm/m^2) – or fractional area change ≤ 33% **By MRI:** • Regional RV akinesia or dyskinesia or dyssynchronous RV contraction • *and* one of the following: – Ratio of RV end-diastolic volume to BSA ≥ 110 mL/m^2 (male) or ≥ 100 mL/m^2 (female) – *or* RV ejection traction ≤ 40% **By RV angiography:** • Regional RV akinesia, dyskinesia, or aneurysm
MINOR	• Mild global RV dilation and/or ejection traction reduction with normal LV • Mild segmental dilation of the RV • Regional RV hepokinesia	**By 2D echo:** • Regional RV akinesia or dyskinesia • *and* one of the following (end diastole): – PLAX RVOT ≥ 29 to < 32 mm (corrected for body size [PLAX/BSA] ≥ 16 to < 19 mm/m^2) – PSAX RVOT ≥ 32 to < 36 mm (corrected for body size [PSAX/BSA] ≥ 18 to < 21 mm/m^2) – *or* fractional area change > 33% to ≤ 40% **By MRI:** • Regional RV akinesia or dyskinesia or dyssynchronous RV contraction • *and* one of the following: – Ratio of RV end-diastolic volume to BSA ≥ 100 to < 110 mL/m^2 (male) or ≥ 90 to < 100 mL/m^2 (female) – *or* RV ejection traction > 40% to ≤ 45%

The combination of a regional RV wall motion abnormality such as akinesia or dyskinesia or the presence of a RV aneurysm with either a dilatation of RVOT or a reduction of RV fractional area change is required for a major criterion. When similar but less pronounced alterations are present, a minor criterion is identified. Source: Modified from Marcus FI, McKenna WJ, Sherrill D, et al.[4]

been described, in clinical practice many physicians rely on visual estimation to assess its size and function.[14] For the diagnosis of ARVC/D, this is certainly not sufficient, because some exact quantifications form an important part of the Task Force Criteria. Thus, the following considerations refer to quantitative aspects of RV size and function as far as the parameters appear in the Task Force Criteria.

Regional Akinesia, Dyskinesia, or Aneurysm

An akinetic segment exhibits neither thickening nor inward movement during systole, while a dyskinetic segment displays no thickening and moves outward during this phase of the cardiac cycle. It is relatively simple to distinguish both of these alterations from normokinetic segments, which show thickening and inward movement during systole. In contrast to the original criteria, hypokinesia is no longer part of the revised Task Force Criteria. As the myocardium of the RV is thinner than that of the LV and the direction of systolic movement is known to be affected by the complex ventricular shape, it may be more difficult to distinguish hypokinesia from other forms of contraction in the RV.[15] Therefore, it is certainly reasonable to exclude hypokinesia from the list of criteria applied for the diagnosis of ARVC/D.

A ventricular aneurysm is defined as a localized, outward bulging of the ventricular wall without any discontinuity of the latter.[16] Diagnosis of an aneurysm is usually straightforward; however, in some instances, it may be difficult to evaluate it in the RV apical region depending on whether the view has been foreshortened. In ARVC/D, multiple ventricular aneurysms can frequently be observed (Figures 6A.2–6A.4).

Right Ventricular Outflow Tract Dimensions

The right ventricle dilates when it starts to fail.[17] The RVOT is best viewed from parasternal and subcostal windows, but it can also be evaluated from the apical window in thin individuals or adults with large intercostal spaces. The modified Task Force Criteria define an upper normal limit for the dimensions of the RVOT in the parasternal long and short axes. The minor criteria for echocardiography were selected at the values at which specificity and sensitivity were equal, while the major criteria were selected at the values that yielded 95% specificity.[4]

Although it is very helpful to have such clearly defined criteria, it is not a simple task to measure the dimensions of the RVOT.[18-20] Even when the aortic valve is taken as a landmark for orientation of the echocardiographic view, it is difficult to exclude oblique images, leading to overestimation of RVOT size. Moreover, the endocardial definition of the anterior wall is often suboptimal.[4] In addition to these technical pitfalls, limited normative data are available, and the window for RVOT size has not been standardized. It is particularly important to realize that the current guidelines for the echocardiographic assessment of the right heart recommend measuring the distal diameter of the RVOT, because this diameter shows the best reproducibility.[4] Unfortunately, the distal diameter is not identical with the diameters included in the revised Task Force Criteria. Finally, the upper limit of the normal range for the RVOT diameters in parasternal long and short axes are not identical in the current guidelines and the revised Task Force Criteria. Certainly, more research is required to solve these important issues.

Right Ventricular Systolic Function

RV systolic function by fractional area change is included in the revised Task Force Criteria.[4] This parameter is determined in the apical 4-chamber view and reflects the percentage change in RV area occurring during systole. This parameter displays a good correlation with measurements derived from magnetic resonance imaging.[21,22] Fractional area change only assesses the dimensions of the RV in a single imaging plane passing through the septum and the lateral free wall, and neither the inflow nor the outflow tract is considered with this measurement. This problem results from the complex geometry of the RV and cannot be solved by a biplanar approach like that applied to the left ventricle; it can only be avoided by a 3D assessment of RV volume.[23-25] Although fractional area change reflects only part of RV systolic function, it is a very useful parameter, since it provides prognostic information in patients with ARVC/D[26] as well as in those with pulmonary embolism[27] and myocardial infarc-

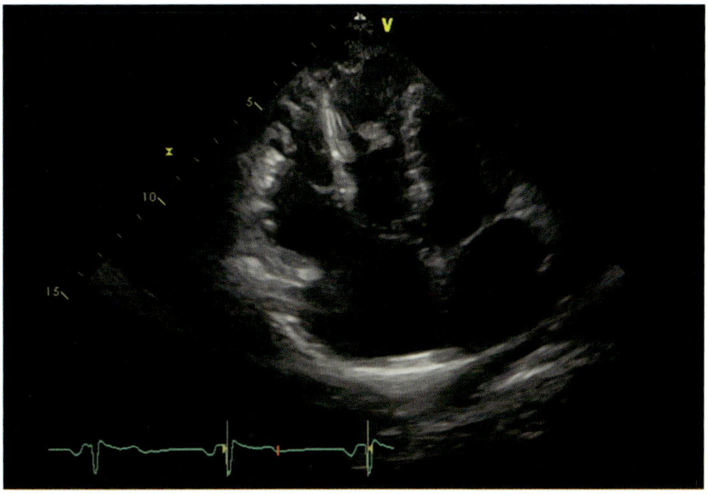

FIGURE 6A.2 Echocardiographic image (modified apical 4-chamber view) of the right ventricle in a patient with ARVC/D diagnosed according to the revised Task Force Criteria.[4] The right ventricle is dilated, and several aneurysms are detectable in the midventricular and apical lateral wall. The reverberating structure in the center of the right ventricle is an ICD electrode.

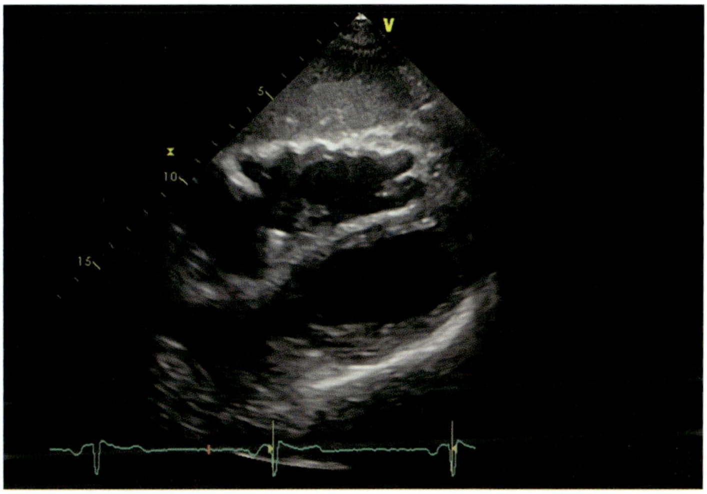

FIGURE 6A.3 Echocardiographic image (subcostal view) of the right ventricle from a patient with ARVC/D diagnosed according to the revised Task Force Criteria.[4] The right ventricle is dilated, and several aneurysms are detectable in the midventricular and apical inferolateral wall.

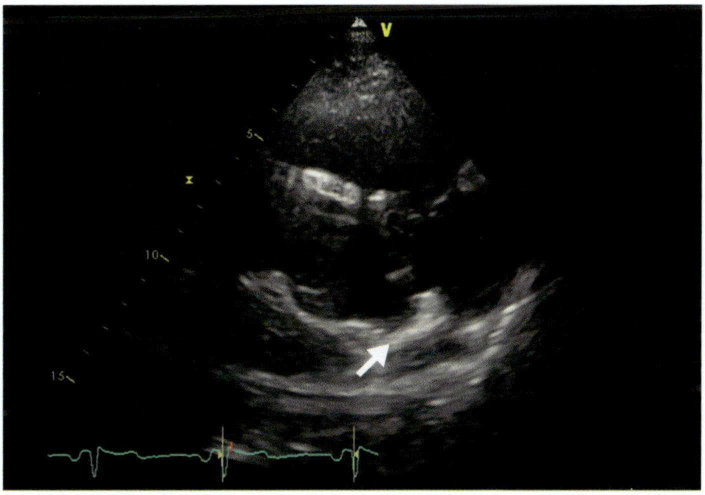

FIGURE 6A.4 Echocardiographic image (modified parasternal long-axis view) of the right ventricle from a patient with ARVC/D diagnosed according to the revised Task Force Criteria.[4] The right ventricle is dilated, and a large aneurysm (**arrow**) is detectable in the subtricuspid area. The reverberating structure in the center of the right ventricle is an ICD electrode.

tion.[28,29] Therefore, at present, fractional area change seems to be an excellent parameter for assessing RV function in patients with ARVC/D.

Another widely used parameter for RV systolic function is tricuspid annulus plane systolic excursion (TAPSE). This parameter reflects the systolic movement of the basal and adjacent segments of the RV wall in the apical 4-chamber view and thus measures the longitudinal systolic function of the RV. The movement of the right ventricle underlying TAPSE is visibly obvious, can easily be measured, and is very reproducible.[30-32] However, it reflects RV systolic function in an even more restricted manner than fractional area change, and one intuitively assumes that it may therefore be of lower value in diseases like ARVC/D, which induces focal myocardial alterations in many patients. A recent study indeed confirmed that the prognostic value of TAPSE is clearly lower than that of fractional area change in patients with ARVC/D.[26]

Future Developments in Echocardiographic Assessment of ARVC/D

Right Ventricular Size

The size of the RV would represent a meaningful parameter in the evaluation of ARVC/D. Although RV size is often compared with that of the LV for a qualitative evaluation,[33] this approach is not sufficient in the context of ARVC/D. A 2D assessment of RV size, as it is performed with different RVOT diameters and with fractional area change, has its limitations as well. Indeed, many parameters of RV size have only recently been evaluated in a large, normal population assessed according to gender and indexed to body surface area.[34] The best assessment of RV size is 3D echocardiography, which allows determination of the volume of the RV more accurately than any other echocardiographic method.[35,36] Indeed, 3D measurements of RV size are less prone to underestimation of the true size than 2D assessment.[37] Boundary tracing errors remain the largest source of error; in addition, it may be difficult to acquire a 3D dataset of the RV that includes its outflow tract, since the latter is located in an anterior position and is often obscured by near-field artifacts. While there are limited normative data available at this time, and the data were only obtained in small series with different methods,[4] 3D measurement of RV size will certainly become an indispensible tool for the echocardiographic evaluation of ARVC/D in the near future.

Right Ventricular Function

Tissue Doppler imaging allows measurement of RV systolic and diastolic function by determining myocardial velocities.[38] Instead of TAPSE, longitudinal function of the RV can be determined by tissue Doppler imaging of the tricuspid annulus. A retrospective study in a small patient group demonstrated a decline of systolic tissue velocity in the RV lateral wall in patients with ARVC/D over time,[39] while another study observed a wide variation of tissue velocity measurements in such patients.[40]

The myocardial performance index (also called Tei index) is a quantitative method for assessing RV function, which is also feasible in many patients with poor image quality.[41] It is calculated as the sum of the isovolumic contraction time and the isovolumic relaxation time divided by the RV ejection time.[42] It has been established that this index is more or less unaffected by heart rate, loading conditions, or tricuspid regurgitation. The value of the Tei index in patients with ARVC/D is yet unknown.

Strain is defined as the degree of deformation of an object, whereas strain rate represents the speed at which strain occurs.[43] Both parameters can be determined by tissue

Doppler imaging. RV longitudinal strain can easily be assessed from the apical view in routine echocardiography.[44] In normal subjects, RV longitudinal velocities are higher than those of the LV and show a baso-apical gradient with higher velocities at the base.[45] This can be explained by the differences in loading conditions with a lower afterload in the right ventricle and by the dominance of longitudinal and oblique myocardial fibers in the RV free wall. Moreover, compared to the homogenous distribution of LV deformation properties, RV strain and strain rate values have an inhomogeneous distribution, which is related to the complex geometry of the thin-walled, crescent-shaped RV compared to the thick-walled, bullet-shaped LV.

Tissue Doppler imaging is an interesting approach for the assessment of regional myocardial function. However, its clinical application may be challenging due to the angle dependence of the currently available tissue Doppler techniques. Due to its complex geometry, this is a particularly important problem in the RV. A new approach to the measurement of strain and strain rate uses frame-by-frame tracking of defined myocardial speckles; the location of the speckles can be tracked on sequential images, and strain data can be generated over the entire chamber. This technology is not angle-dependent and may represent a considerable advantage for analysis of the RV.[46] It can also be used in a 3D manner, and thus opens new possibilities to analyze the complexity of RV function in a more appropriate manner.[47] A recent study applied speckle-derived myocardial strain for assessing RV mechanical dispersion, observed that the latter was more pronounced in ARVC/D patients with ventricular tachyarrhythmias, and suggested that this method might be used for risk stratification in asymptomatic mutation carriers.[48]

These methodological developments indicate that echocardiography will still play an important role for the diagnosis of ARVC/D in the next decade. Indeed, physicians have just started to apply the new technologies mentioned above, in particular 3D imaging of the RV, in clinical routine.

Abbreviations

ICD implantable cardioverter-defibrillator
LV left ventricle, left ventricular
RV right ventricle
RVOT right ventricular outflow tract
TAPSE tricuspid annulus plane systolic excursion

References

1. Basso C, Corrado D, Marcus FI, Nava A, Thiene G. Arrhythmogenic right ventricular cardiomyopathy. *Lancet.* 2009;373:1289-1300.
2. Corrado D, Basso C, Thiene G, et al. Spectrum of clinicopathologic manifestation of arrhythmogenic right ventricular cardiomyopathy/dysplasia: a multicenter study. *J Am Coll Cardiol.* 1997;6:1512-1520.
3. McKenna WJ, Thiene G, Nava A, et al, on behalf of the Task Force of the Working Group Myocardial and Pericardial Disease of the European Society of Cardiology and of the Scientific Council on Cardiomyopathies of the International Society and Federation of Cardiology. Diagnosis of arrhythmogenic right ventricular dysplasia cardiomyopathy. *Br Heart J.* 1994;71:215-218.
4. Marcus FI, McKenna WJ, Sherrill D, et al. Diagnosis of arrhythmogenic right ventricular cardiomyopathy/dysplasia: proposed modification of the Task Force Criteria. *Circulation.* 2010;121:1533-1541.
5. Thiene G, Corrado D, Basso C. Arrhythmogenic right ventricular cardiomyopathy/dysplasia. *Orphanet J Rare Dis.* 2007;14(2):45-61.
6. Marra MP, Leoni L, Bauce B, et al. Imaging study of ventricular scar in arrhythmogenic right ventricular cardiomyopathy: comparison of 3D standard electroanatomical voltage mapping and contrast-enhanced cardiac magnetic resonance. *Circ Arrhythm Electrophysiol.* 2012;5:91-100.

7. Rizzo S, Pilichou K, Thiene G, Basso C. The changing spectrum of arrhythmogenic (right ventricular) cardiomyopathy. *Cell Tissue Res.* 2012;348:319-323.
8. Kisslo J. Two-dimensional echocardiography in arrhythmogenic right ventricular dysplasia. *Eur Heart J.* 1989;10(Suppl D):22-26.
9. Pinamonti B, Dragos AM, Pyxaras SA, et al. Prognostic predictors in arrhythmogenic right ventricular cardiomyopathy: results from a 10-year registry. *Eur Heart J.* 2011;32:1105-1113.
10. Teske AJ, Cox MG, Te Riele AS, et al. Early detection of regional functional abnormalities in asymptomatic ARVD/C gene carriers. *J Am Soc Echocardiogr.* 2012;25:997-1006.
11. Forman MB, Goodin J, Phelan B, Kopelman H, Virmani R. Electrocardiographic changes associated with isolated right ventricular infarction. *J Am Coll Cardiol.* 1984;4:640-643.
12. Ho SY, Nihoyannopoulos P. Anatomy, echocardiography, and normal right ventricular dimensions. *Heart.* 2006;92:i2-i13.
13. Lang RM, Bierig M, Devereux RB, Flachskampf FA, Foster E, Pellikka PA. Recommendations for chamber quantification: a report from the American Society of Echocardiography's Guidelines and Standards Committee and the Chamber Quantification Writing Group, developed in conjunction with the European Association of Echocardiography, a branch of the European Society of Cardiology. *J Am Soc Echocardiogr.* 2005;18:1440-1463.
14. Rudski LG, Lai WW, Afilalo J, et al. Guidelines for the echocardiographic assessment of the right heart in adults: a report from the American Society of Echocardiography endorsed by the European Association of Echocardiography, a registered branch of the European Society of Cardiology, and the Canadian Society of Echocardiography. *J Am Soc Echocardiogr.* 2010;23:685-713.
15. Vermes E, Strohm O, Otmani A, Childs H, Duff H, Friedrich MG. Impact of the revision of arrhythmogenic right ventricular cardiomyopathy/dysplasia Task Force Criteria on its prevalence by CMR criteria. *JACC Cardiovasc Imaging.* 2011;4:282-287.
16. Zoffoli G, Mangino D, Venturini A, et al. Diagnosing left ventricular aneurysm from pseudo-aneurysm: a case report and a review in literature. *J Cardiothorac Surg.* 2009;4:11-16.
17. Haddad F, Doyle R, Murphy DJ, Hunt SA. Right ventricular function in cardiovascular disease, part II: pathophysiology, clinical importance, and management of right ventricular failure. *Circulation.* 2008;117:1717-1731.
18. Bashore TM. Adult congenital heart disease: right ventricular outflow tract lesions. *Circulation.* 2007;115:1933-1947.
19. Yoerger DM, Marcus F, Sherrill D, et al. Multidisciplinary Study of Right Ventricular Dysplasia Investigators. Echocardiographic findings in patients meeting Task Force Criteria for arrhythmogenic right ventricular dysplasia: new insights from the multidisciplinary study of right ventricular dysplasia. *J Am Coll Cardiol.* 2005;45:860-865.
20. Anwar AM, Soliman O, van den Bosch AE, et al. Assessment of pulmonary valve and right ventricular outflow tract with real-time three-dimensional echocardiography. *Int J Cardiovasc Imaging.* 2007;23:167-175.
21. Lai WW, Gauvreau K, Rivera ES, Saleeb S, Powell AJ, Geva T. Accuracy of guideline recommendations for two-dimensional quantification of the right ventricle by echocardiography. *Int J Cardiovasc Imaging.* 2008;24:691-698.
22. Anavekar NS, Gerson D, Skali H, Kwong RY, Yucel EK, Solomon SD. Two-dimensional assessment of right ventricular function: an echocardiographic-MRI correlative study. *Echocardiography.* 2007;24:452-456.
23. Linker DT, Moritz WE, Pearlman AS. A new three-dimensional echocardiographic method of right ventricular volume measurement: in vitro validation. *J Am Coll Cardiol.* 1986;8:101-106.
24. Schindera ST, Mehwald PS, Sahn DJ, Kececioglu D. Accuracy of real-time three-dimensional echocardiography for quantifying right ventricular volume: static and pulsatile flow studies in an anatomic in vitro model. *J Ultrasound Med.* 2002;21:1069-1075.
25. Grison A, Maschietto N, Reffo E, et al. Three-dimensional echocardiographic evalu-

ation of right ventricular volume and function in pediatric patients: validation of the technique. *J Am Soc Echocardiogr.* 2007;20: 921-929.

26. Saguner AM, Vecchiati A, Baldinger SH, et al. Different Prognostic Value of Functional Right Ventricular Parameters in Arrhythmogenic Right Ventricular Cardiomyopathy/Dysplasia. *Circ Cardiovasc Imaging.* 2014;7(2):230-239.
27. Nass N, McConnell MV, Goldhaber SZ, Chyu S, Solomon SD. Recovery of regional right ventricular function after thrombolysis for pulmonary embolism. *Am J Cardiol.* 1999;83:804-806.
28. Zornoff LA, Skali H, Pfeffer MA, et al. Right ventricular dysfunction and risk of heart failure and mortality after myocardial infarction. *J Am Coll Cardiol.* 2002;39:1450-1445.
29. Anavekar NS, Skali H, Bourgoun M, et al. Usefulness of right ventricular fractional area change to predict death, heart failure, and stroke following myocardial infarction (from the VALIANT ECHO study). *Am J Cardiol.* 2008;101:607-612.
30. Kaul S, Tei C, Hopkins JM, Shah PM. Assessment of right ventricular function using two-dimensional echocardiography. *Am Heart J.* 1984;107:526-531.
31. Lopez-Candales A, Dohi K, Rajagopalan N, Edelman K, Gulyasy B, Bazaz R. Defining normal variables of right ventricular size and function in pulmonary hypertension: an echocardiographic study. *Postgrad Med J.* 2008;84:40-45.
32. Miller D, Farah MG, Liner A, Fox K, Schluchter M, Hoit BD. The relation between quantitative right ventricular ejection fraction and indices of tricuspid annular motion and myocardial performance. *J Am Soc Echocardiogr.* 2004;17:443-447.
33. Vitarelli A, Terzano C. Do we have two hearts? New insights in right ventricular function supported by myocardial imaging echocardiography. *Heart Fail Rev.* 2010;15:39-61.
34. D'Oronzio U, Senn O, Biaggi P, et al. Right heart assessment by echocardiography: gender and body size matters. *J Am Soc Echocardiogr.* 2012;25:1251-1258.
35. Nesser HJ, Tkalec W, Patel AR, et al. Quantitation of right ventricular volumes and ejection fraction by three-dimensional echocardiography in patients: comparison with magnetic resonance imaging and radionuclide ventriculography. *Echocardiography.* 2006;23:666-680.
36. Horton KD, Meece RW, Hill JC. Assessment of the right ventricle by echocardiography: a primer for cardiac sonographers. *J Am Soc Echocardiogr.* 2009;22:776-792.
37. Jenkins C, Chan J, Bricknell K, Strudwick M, Marwick TH. Reproducibility of right ventricular volumes and ejection fraction using real-time three-dimensional echocardiography: comparison with cardiac MRI. *Chest.* 2007;131:1844-1851.
38. Kukulski T, Hübbert L, Arnold M, Wranne B, Hatle L, Sutherland GR. Normal regional right ventricular function and its change with age: a Doppler myocardial imaging study. *J Am Soc Echocardiogr.* 2000;13:194-204.
39. Aneq MÅ, Lindström L, Fluur C, Nylander E. Long-term follow-up in arrhythmogenic right ventricular cardiomyopathy using tissue Doppler imaging. *Scand Cardiovasc J.* 2008;42:368-374.
40. Kjaergaard J, Hastrup Svendsen J, Sogaard P, et al. Advanced quantitative echocardiography in arrhythmogenic right ventricular cardiomyopathy. *J Am Soc Echocardiogr.* 2007;20:27-35.
41. Tei C, Dujardin KS, Hodge DO, et al. Doppler echocardiographic index for assessment of global right ventricular function. *J Am Soc Echocardiogr.* 1996;9:838-847.
42. Burgess MI, Bright-Thomas RJ, Ray SG. Echocardiographic evaluation of right ventricular function. *Eur J Echocardiogr.* 2002;3:252-262.
43. Kowalski M, Kukulski T, Jamal F, et al. Can natural strain and strain rate quantify regional myocardial deformation? A study in healthy subjects. *Ultrasound Med Biol.* 2001;27:1087-1097.
44. Pettersen E, Helle-Valle T, Edvardsen T, et al. Contraction pattern of the systemic right ventricle shift from longitudinal to circumferential shortening and absent global ventricular torsion. *J Am Coll Cardiol.* 2007;49: 2450-2456.

45. Gondi S, Dokainish H. Right ventricular tissue Doppler and strain imaging: ready for clinical use? *Echocardiography.* 2007;24: 522-532.
46. Aneq MÅ, Engvall J, Brudin L, Nylander E. Evaluation of right and left ventricular function using speckle tracking echocardiography in patients with arrhythmogenic right ventricular cardiomyopathy and their first degree relatives. *Cardiovasc Ultrasound.* 2012;10:37.
47. Atsumi A, Ishizu T, Kameda Y, et al. Application of 3-dimensional speckle tracking imaging to the assessment of right ventricular regional deformation. *Circ J.* 2013;77:1760-1768.
48. Sarvari SI, Haugaa KH, Anfinsen OG, et al. Right ventricular mechanical dispersion is related to malignant arrhythmias: a study of patients with arrhythmogenic right ventricular cardiomyopathy and subclinical right ventricular dysfunction. *Eur Heart J.* 2011;32: 1089-1096.

6B

The Role of Cardiac Magnetic Resonance Imaging in Arrhythmogenic Right Ventricular Cardiomyopathy/Dysplasia

Robert Manka, MD, and Markus Niemann, MD

Introduction

The 2010 International Task Force Criteria[1] call for a thorough cardiac imaging evaluation of patients with arrhythmogenic right ventricular cardiomyopathy/dysplasia (ARVC/D). Cardiac magnetic resonance (CMR) is widely acknowledged as the standard for cardiac mass and volume analysis.[2-5] Moreover, since the first-line diagnostic tool, echocardiography, might be cumbersome when it comes to the assessment of the right ventricle (RV)[6] due to acoustic window dependency, incomplete visualization of the RV in all echocardiographic views, and geometric assumptions, CMR plays an important role in diagnosing patients with ARVC/D.[7] This is supported by the possibility that an acquired 3D dataset can be sampled in any plane using CMR, and a serial evaluation of the same patient over time can easily be performed (Figure 6B.1).

Although CMR offers great diagnostic facilities, limitations and challenges with this technique must not be left aside.[8] When ARVC/D came into clinicians' field of view in the late 1980s, CMR was in its infancy.[9-11] Although the disease has ever since been associated with the substitution of RV myocardium by fibrofatty infiltrations,[10,12] the role of CMR was not clearly defined by the first Task Force Criteria published in 1994.[13] Because the new Task Force Criteria in 2010 eliminated the criterion of noninvasive detection of fat and clearly defined CMR criteria for ARVC/D based on regional wall motion abnormalities, RV volumes, and RV function,[1] some ARVC/D patient cohorts should be revisited. Nevertheless, the possibility to characterize tissue using CMR provides information that cannot be gathered that easily using other noninvasive tests.[10,14] Therefore, CMR might have taken over the leading role in imaging diagnostics from the former gold standard angiography in ARVC/D justly.

Current Concepts in Arrhythmogenic Right Ventricular Cardiomyopathy/Dysplasia
© 2014 Corinna Brunckhorst and Firat Duru, Editors. Cardiotext Publishing, ISBN: 978-1-935395-92-8

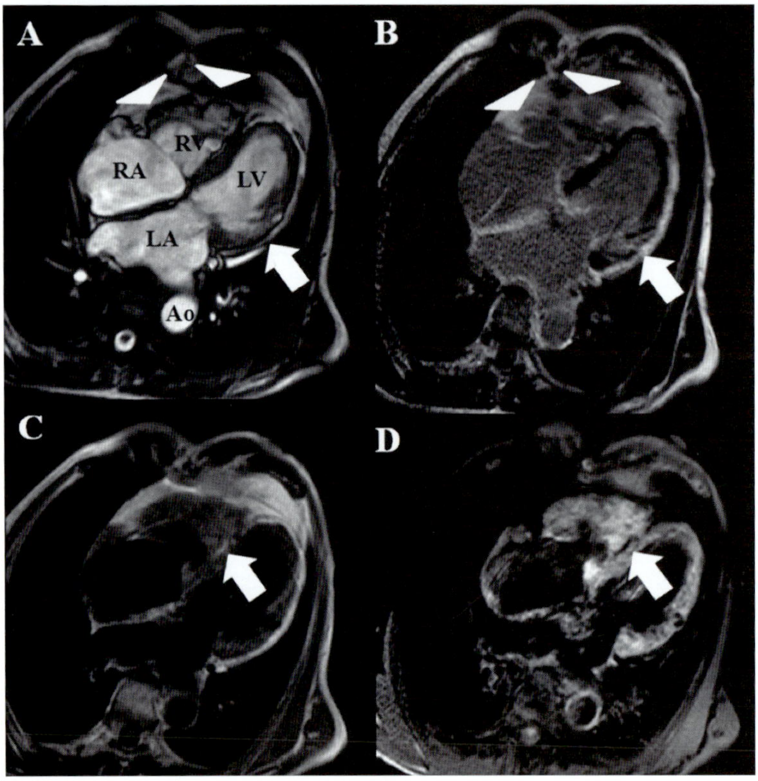

FIGURE 6B.1 Cardiac magnetic resonance (CMR) imaging in a male patient with arrhythmogenic right ventricular cardiomyopathy (ARVC/D) and extensive left ventricular involvement. **Panel A:** Cine images show abnormalities of regional and global right ventricular (**white arrow heads**) and left ventricular (**white arrow**) function. The right atrium (RA) is also dilated. **Panel B:** Late enhancement images confirm extensive fibrosis of the RV free wall (**white arrow heads**) and LV lateral wall (**white arrow**). T1-weighted images without (**Panel C**) and with (**Panel D**) fat suppression demonstrate fatty infiltrations (**white arrow**) of the interventricular septum. Ao = Aorta; LA = left atrium; LV = left ventricle; RA = right atrium; RV = right ventricle.

Major and Minor CMR Criteria of ARVC/D

The Task Force Criteria for CMR, first published in 1994,[13] have been revised grossly in the new version in 2010.[1] The changes were mainly made because the 1994 Task Force Criteria had high specificity and lacked sensitivity—thus, early stages might have been missed using the original criteria.[1,15] However, several reports and cohorts have been published since 1994 that relied very much on CMR tissue characterization (proof of myocardial fat), and thus, some patients might have been falsely identified as having ARVC/D. This was shown nicely by a study conducted at the Johns Hopkins Hospital, Baltimore, Maryland.[16] When looking at the new 2010 Task Force Criteria in regard to CMR, most important is the need of the presence of wall motion abnormalities and simultaneous quantitative features of RV alteration (eg, measurements of dimension and function).[1] In addition, the suspicion of fat in a CMR image is not a sufficient feature to fulfill a major or minor criterion. This seems to be reasonable, since Bluemke et al showed that the interobserver variability for the detection of intramyocardial fat is high.[17] Moreover, intramyocardial fat is not specific for ARVC/D but can be found in patients with long-term administration of steroids, elderly patients, in various other conditions including other cardiomyopathies, and also even in healthy subjects.[18-20]

The major and minor criteria for imaging in the 2010 Task Force Criteria are as follows:

- *Major:* Regional RV akinesia or dyskinesia or dyssynchronus RV contraction and one of the following:

  - ratio of the RV end-diastolic volume to body surface area (BSA) $\geq$ 110 mL/m^2 (male) or $\geq$ 100 mL/m^2 (female) or
  - RV ejection fraction $\leq$ 40%

- *Minor*: Regional RV akinesia or dyskinesia or dyssynchronus RV contraction and one of the following:
  - ratio of the RV end-diastolic volume to BSA $\geq$ 100 mL/m^2 to < 110 mL/m^2 (male) or $\geq$ 90 mL/m^2 to < 100 mL/m^2 (female) or
  - RV ejection fraction > 40% to $\leq$ 45%

In early stages, the wall motion abnormalities might be confined to the subtricuspid region, the RV outflow tract (RVOT), and later the RV apex (the so-called triangle of dysplasia).[11] However, the preference for these localizations has recently been questioned by Dr. Calkins and Dr. Tandri from Johns Hopkins, since in their experience, the RV apex is involved at very late stages of the disease.Minor, regional wall motion abnormalities such as hypokinesia at the insertion of the moderator band are often part of the normal spectrum.[1,21] Hypokinesia is commonly defined as a thickening of no more than 40% during systole and akinesia as a thickening of no more than 10% during systole. The analysis of RV mechanics can be supported using CMR tagging.[22]

Establishing the RV volume as a red flag is supported by a study of Ma et al, who investigated 40 patients with ARVC/D to evaluate the relationship between CMR abnormalities and QRS dispersion.[23] QRS dispersion is regarded as an electrocardiographic independent predictor of sudden death in patients with ARVC/D. The authors could show that the RVOT area and the RV end-diastolic and end-systolic volumes were positively correlated to the extent of QRS dispersion in their cohort.[23]

Additional Morphological Features

Like intramyocardial fat, wall thinning, trabecular disarray, or late gadolinium enhancement (LGE), which can be of potential help when characterizing the RV in patients with ARVC/D, are no longer mentioned in the current Task Force Criteria.[1]

Wall Thinning and Hypertrophy

Although its prevalence varies, wall thinning due to fatty infiltration and loss/replacement of myocardial tissue seems to be a more common finding than RV hypertrophy in patients with ARVC/D.[24,25]

Trabeculae

Similar to other RV pathologies presenting with ventricular dilatation, in up to half of ARVC/D patients, a prominent trabeculation can be found.[25]

Right Ventricular Outflow Tract

The dimension of the RVOT is an echocardiographic criterion for ARVC/D.[1] In CMR, this criterion is not used; however, the practitioner should think of ARVC/D when a dilated and dysmorphed RVOT is seen on CMR images.

Fibrosis

The substitution of myocardial tissue in ARVC/D is not only due to fat, but rather combined fibrofatty infiltration. Thus, LGE imaging might reveal valuable information in patients with suspected and confirmed ARVC/D. Gadolinium, the contrast agent used in LGE imaging, is unable to cross the cell membrane; in the presence of scar/fibrosis, gadolinium accumulates in areas with extended extracellular space and affects relaxation times, leading to hyperenhancement in T1-weighted images. While initial ex vivo studies used a signal intensity of 2–3 standard deviations above the normal-appearing myocardium in order to detect LGE, newer studies have used up to 6 standard deviations in vivo (due to motion and blurring) and alternatively a threshold > 50% of the maximal signal intensity within the scar.[26-29] In a study by Tandri et al, there was an excellent correlation between CMR, LGE findings, and histopathology in their ARVC/D cohort.[17] The regions of fibrosis should match with the hypo- and akinetic regions on cine images. Moreover, a differentiation between ARVC/D and idiopathic ventricular tachycardia from the RVOT might be supported by LGE imaging, because patients with idiopathic RVOT tachycardia should not show fibrosis on CMR—although this is not a *sine qua non* criterion (Figure 6B.2).

ARVC/D patients with fibrosis show a higher susceptibility to arrhythmias than patients without LGE. Although this suggests that inducibility of malignant ventricular tachycardias correlates with regions of LGE, there are no studies directly investigating the arrhythmogenic substrate in patients with ARVC/D.[26] This might be because of the thinner RV wall compared to the left ventricular (LV) wall, which promotes misdelineation of the borders of myocardial tissue. Moreover, the so-called Look-Locker sequences (nulling of the myocardium to detect LGE) is done using the LV, which might result in wrong timing for the RV.

Power and Benefit of CMR Imaging in ARVC/D

CMR can reveal information about functional and morphological alterations in patients with ARVC/D, which is facilitated by advances in CMR technology in recent years, including better and faster imaging acquisition methods (steady-state free-precession [SSFP] imaging, black blood imaging). In contrast to echocardiography, CMR can also visualize the tissue surrounding the heart, revealing pathologies that might mimic ARVC/D, such as thoracic abnormalities (eg, pectus excavatum) or abnormal heart positions with concomitant distortion of RV shape (eg, partially absent pericardium).[21] Special ARVC/D CMR protocols exist, which are mainly based on SSFP-cine, T1-weighted black blood, T1-weighted black blood with fat suppression, and LGE imaging.

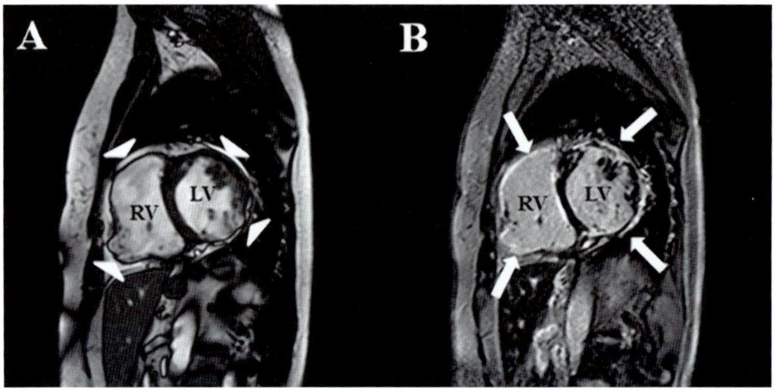

FIGURE 6B.2 Cardiac magnetic resonance (CMR) imaging in a 60-year-old female patient with arrhythmogenic right ventricular cardiomyopathy (ARVC/D) and extensive left ventricular involvement. **Panel A:** End-systolic short-axis cine image shows abnormalities of regional and global right ventricular (RV) and left ventricular (LV) function (**white arrow heads**). **Panel B:** Late enhancement images confirm extensive fibrosis of the RV and LV walls (**white arrows**).

Cine Imaging

Cine imaging is used to quantify RV function. Signal intensity in SSFP sequences is not affected by reduction in flowing blood velocity in cases of dysfunctional RV as compared to gradient echo imaging sequences.[7] In addition to the standard short-axis, 2-chamber, 4-chamber, and 3-chamber views, SSFP-cine sequences of the RVOT, the RV 2-chamber, and the RV transversal view should be acquired.

T1-Weighted Black Blood Imaging

T1-weighted black blood imaging in ARVC/D is performed routinely as black blood images with double-inversion-recovery, fast spin-echo sequences during breath-hold.[30] These sequences improve contrast and reduce motion artifacts in comparison to traditional spin-echo sequences. On black blood images, fat appears hyperintense. In healthy volunteers, epicardial fat can be clearly demarcated from the RV myocardium. The gross amount of epicardial fat can be found at the RV free wall, as well as in the interventricular and atrioventricular grooves. In patients with ARVC/D, there might be streaks of fat that originate from the epicardial fat and infiltrate the RV myocardium. Different studies suggest varying prevalences of fatty infiltration visualized by CMR. With highly sensitive protocols and advanced CMR techniques, up to 75% of ARVC/D patients might present fatty infiltrations of the RV.[25] Schick et al could show that chemical shift selective sequences improve tissue characterization and fat and fibrosis delineation.[31]

The same T1-weighted black blood sequences described above should also be performed using fat suppression (eg, STIR).

Differential Diagnosis of ARVC/D

There has been some discussion whether myocarditis might mimic ARVC/D in some cases.[32,33] A study by Pieroni et al suggested that 3D electroanatomical mapping-guided endomyocardial biopsy might be able to differentiate these 2 entities.[33] However, perfect mimicry of ARVC/D by myocarditis seems to be a rather rare finding.[32]

Myocardial sarcoidosis and ARVC/D share more common features, as we also know from autopsy studies. This seems to be especially true for the left ventricular "type" of arrhythmogenic cardiomyopathy (see below).[34] Some changes in RV structure similar to that observed in ARVC/D have been reported in patients with Brugada syndrome by Catalano et al.[35] In addition, the absence of pericardium around the RV may mimic aneurysms and wall motion abnormalities found in ARVC/D patients. Another important issue is the differentiation between early manifestations of ARVC/D and the athlete's heart. An early report by Corrado et al suggested a high prevalence of ARVC/D in suddenly deceased highly competitive athletes.[36] Luijkx et al could demonstrate that a simple left-to-right end-diastolic volume index (LV/RV EDV ratio) can be of value to differentiate the athlete's heart from patients with ARVC/D.[37] The athlete's heart shows a proportionate adaptation of the RV and the LV and thus a significantly lower RV/LV EDV ratio (close to the controls—value of around 1.1) in contrast to patients with ARVC/D (ratio of 1.4).[37] Also clinically important is the differentiation between ARVC/D and idiopathic RVOT tachycardia. In addition to the aforementioned characteristics, which can be worked out using CMR, Tandri et al showed that it might be possible to differentiate patients with ARVC/D from those with idiopathic RVOT tachycardia by performing 3D electroanatomical mapping using endocardial activation duration,[38] which was significantly prolonged in patients with ARVC/D.[38] Moreover, patients with idiopathic RVOT tachycardia do not display prolonged signal duration and areas of low voltage. A special cardiomyopathy called Uhl's anomaly is characterized by a paper-thin RV, caused by an almost complete absence of myocardial fibers; thus, ARVC/D might be misdiagnosed in some cases.[39,40]

Left-Sided Arrhythmogenic Cardiomyopathy

In the 1994 Task Force Criteria, it was stated that only mild LV dysfunction should be present in patients with ARVC/D, and that LV involvement should preferably occur at late stages of the disease. However, more recent reports have described advanced biventricular and early LV involvement. Pinamonti et al reported a 23-year-old male patient with biventricular involvement where the postmortem specimen revealed fatty infiltrations in the RV and LV. This was also shown on postmortem CMR images. In a small study of 6 ARVC/D patients, 2 presented LGE in the LV.[41] LV involvement in different ARVC/D cohorts seems to vary quite remarkably, from 16% to 76%.[42,43] Even a left-dominant type of arrhythmogenic cardiomyopathy is being discussed. Most commonly, the posterolateral region of the LV is affected; a nicely illustrative case was reported by Paetsch et al.[44] This might lead to the conclusion that neither predominant RV or LV involvement represents distinct cardiomyopathies, but patterns of a generalized arrhythmogenic cardiomyopathy.[43] This is supported by the fact that ARVC/D is mostly a desmosomal disease, and desmosomes are expressed in both ventricles (Figure 6B.3).

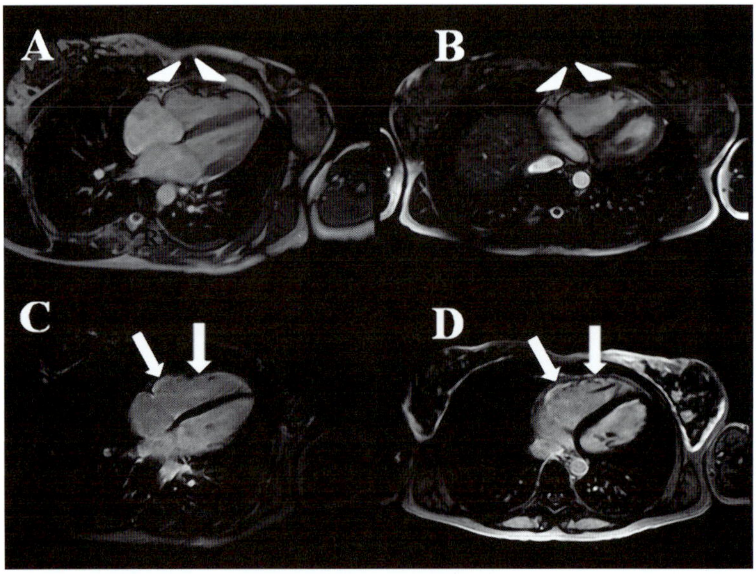

FIGURE 6B.3 Cardiac magnetic resonance (CMR) imaging in a 32-year-old female patient with arrhythmogenic right ventricular cardiomyopathy (ARVC/D). Endsystolic cine 4-chamber (**Panel A**) and axial (**Panel B**) images show regional wall motion abnormalities (**white arrowheads**). **Panels C** and **D:** Late enhancement images confirm extensive fibrosis of the RV wall (**white arrow**).

Conclusion

ARVC/D cannot and must not be diagnosed solely on CMR criteria. Thus, ARVC/D will remain a diagnostic challenge, taking into account that there simply is no gold standard for the diagnosis of ARVC/D. Nevertheless, CMR has become an important and powerful diagnostic tool in the assessment of ARVC/D.

Abbreviations

LV left ventricle, left ventricular
RV right ventricle, right ventricular

References

1. Marcus, FI, McKenna WJ, Sherrill D, et al. Diagnosis of arrhythmogenic right ventricular cardiomyopathy/dysplasia (ARVC/D). *Circulation.* 2010;121(13):1533-1541.
2. Nagueh SF, Bierig SM, Budoff MJ, et al. American Society of Echocardiography clinical recommendations for multimodality cardiovascular imaging of patients with hypertrophic cardiomyopathy: endorsed by the American Society of Nuclear Cardiology, Society for Cardiovascular Magnetic Resonance, and Society of Cardiovascular Computed Tomography. *J Am Soc Echocardiogr.* 2011;24(5):473-498.
3. Lorenz CH, Walker ES, Morgan VL, Klein SS, Graham TP Jr. Normal human right and left ventricular mass, systolic function, and gender differences by cine magnetic resonance imaging. *J Cardiovasc Magn Reson.* 1999;1(1):7-21.
4. Alfakih K, Reid S, Jones T, Sivananthan M. Assessment of ventricular function and mass by cardiac magnetic resonance imaging. *Eur Radiol.* 2004;14(10):1813-1822.
5. Lyne JC, Pennell DJ. Cardiovascular magnetic resonance in the quantitative assessment of left ventricular mass, volumes and contractile function. *Coron Artery Dis.* 2005;16(6):337-343.
6. Armstrong AC, Gidding S, Gjesdal O, Wu C, Bluemke DA, Lima JA. LV mass assessed by echocardiography and CMR, cardiovascular outcomes, and medical practice. *JACC Cardiovasc Imaging.* 2012;5(8):837-848.
7. Jain A, Tandri H, Calkins H, Bluemke DA. Role of cardiovascular magnetic resonance imaging in arrhythmogenic right ventricular dysplasia. *J Cardiovasc Magn Reson.* 2008;10(1):32.
8. Atalay MK. Establishing a cardiac MRI program: problems, pitfalls, expectations. *J Am Coll Radiol.* 2005;2(9):740-748.
9. Fontaine G, Frank R, Tonet JL, et al. Arrhythmogenic right ventricular dysplasia: a clinical model for the study of chronic ventricular tachycardia. *Jpn Circ J.* 1984;48(6):515-538 (1984).
10. Wolf JE, Rose-Pittet L, Page E, et al. Detection of parietal lesions using magnetic resonance imaging in arrhythmogenic dysplasia of the right ventricle. *Arch Mal Coeur Vaiss.* 1989;82(10):1711-1717.
11. Marcus FI, Fontaine GH, Guiraudon G, et al. Right ventricular dysplasia: a report of 24 adult cases. *Circulation.* 1982;65(2):384-398.
12. Molinari G, Sardanelli F, Zandrino F, et al. Adipose replacement and wall motion abnormalities in right ventricle arrhythmias: evaluation by MR imaging. Retrospective evaluation on 124 patients. *Int J Card Imaging.* 2000;16(2):105-115.
13. McKenna WJ, Thiene G, Nava A, et al. Diagnosis of arrhythmogenic right ventricular dysplasia/cardiomyopathy. Task Force of the Working Group Myocardial and Pericardial Disease of the European Society of Cardiology and of the Scientific Council on Cardiomyopathies of the International Society and Federation of Cardiology. *Br Heart J.* 1994;71(3):215-218.
14. Ntusi NA, Francis JM, Matthews PM, et al. Myocardial tissue characterisation with late gadolinium enhancement in rheumatoid arthritis, systemic lupus erythematosus and systemic sclerosis. *J Cardiovasc Magn Reson.* 2013;15(Suppl 1):O47.
15. Antoniades L, Tsatsopoulou A, Anastasakis A, et al. Arrhythmogenic right ventricular cardiomyopathy caused by deletions in plakophilin-2 and plakoglobin (Naxos disease) in families from Greece and Cyprus: genotype–pheno-

type relations, diagnostic features and prognosis. *Eur Heart J.* 2006;27(18):2208-2216.

16. Bomma C, Rutberg J, Tandri H, et al. Misdiagnosis of arrhythmogenic right ventricular dysplasia/cardiomyopathy. *J Cardiovasc Electrophysiol.* 2004;15(3):300-306.
17. Tandri H, Saranathan M, Rodriguez ER, et al. Noninvasive detection of myocardial fibrosis in arrhythmogenic right ventricular cardiomyopathy using delayed-enhancement magnetic resonance imaging. *J Am Coll Cardiol.* 2005;45(1):98-103.
18. Kirsch J, Johansen CK, Araoz PA, Brady PA, Williamson EE, Glockner JF. Prevalence of fat deposition within the right ventricular myocardium in asymptomatic young patients without ventricular arrhythmias. *J Thorac Imaging.* 2010;25(2):173-178.
19. O'Connor S, Recavarren R, Nichols LC, Parwani AV. Lipomatous hypertrophy of the interatrial septum: an overview. *Arch Pathol Lab Med.* 2006;130(3):397-399.
20. Kellman P, Hernando D, Arai AE. Myocardial fat imaging. *Curr Cardiovasc Imaging Rep.* 2010;3(2):83-91.
21. Quarta G, Sado DM, Moon JC. Cardiomyopathies: focus on cardiovascular magnetic resonance. *Br J Radiol.* 2011;84(Spec No 3):S296-S305.
22. Naito H, Arisawa J, Harada K, Yamagami H, Kozuka T, Tamura S. Assessment of right ventricular regional contraction and comparison with the left ventricle in normal humans: a cine magnetic resonance study with presaturation myocardial tagging. *Br Heart J.* 1995;74(2):186-191.
23. Ma N, Cheng H, Lu M, Jiang S, Yin G, Zhao S. Cardiac magnetic resonance imaging in arrhythmogenic right ventricular cardiomyopathy: correlation to the QRS dispersion. *Magn Reson Imaging.* 2012;30(10):1454-1560.
24. White RD, Trohman RG, Flamm SD, et al. Right ventricular arrhythmia in the absence of arrhythmogenic dysplasia: MR imaging of myocardial abnormalities. *Radiology.* 1998;207(3):743-751.
25. Tandri H, Calkins H, Nasir K, et al. Magnetic resonance imaging findings in patients meeting Task Force Criteria for arrhythmogenic right ventricular dysplasia. *J Cardiovasc Electrophysiol.* 2003;14(5):476-482.
26. Yokokawa M, Mueller G, Bogun F. Role of imaging in ablation therapy of ventricular arrhythmias. Focus on cardiac magnetic resonance imaging. *Circ J.* 2012;76(6):1292-1298.
27. Kim RJ, Fieno DS, Parrish TB, et al. Relationship of MRI delayed contrast enhancement to irreversible injury, infarct age, and contractile function. *Circulation* 1999;100:1992-2002.
28. Simonetti OP, Kim RJ, Fieno DS, et al. An improved MR imaging technique for the visualization of myocardial infarction. *Radiology.* 2001;218(1):215-223.
29. Amado LC, Gerber BL, Gupta SN, et al. Accurate and objective infarct sizing by contrast-enhanced magnetic resonance imaging in a canine myocardial infarction model. *J Am Coll Cardiol.* 2004;44(12):2383-2389.
30. Erriquez D, Di Cesare E, Barile A, Gallucci M, Splendiani A, Masciocchi C. Cardiac MRI: comparison between single-shot fast spin echo and conventional spin echo sequences in the morphological evaluation of the ventricles. *Radiol Med.* 2002; 103(1-2):34-44.
31. Schick F, Miller S, Hahn U. Fat- and water-selective MR cine imaging of the human heart: assessment of right ventricular dysplasia. *Invest Radiol.* 2000;35(5):311-318.
32. Thiene G, Basso C, Corrado D. May active myocarditis mimic arrhythmogenic right ventricular cardiomyopathy phenotype by electroanatomic mapping? *J Am Coll Cardiol.* 2009;54(13):1190.
33. Pieroni M, Dello Russo A, Marzo F, et al. High prevalence of myocarditis mimicking arrhythmogenic right ventricular cardiomyopathy: differential diagnosis by electroanatomic mapping-guided endomyocardial biopsy. *J Am Coll Cardiol.* 2009;53(8):681-689.
34. Barbou F, Lahutte M, Gontier E. Cardiac sarcoidosis presenting as an arrhythmogenic right ventricular cardiomyopathy. *Heart.* 2012;98(23):1753-1754.
35. Catalano O, Antonaci S, Moro G, et al. Magnetic resonance investigations in Bru-

gada syndrome reveal unexpectedly high rate of structural abnormalities. *Eur Heart J.* 2009;30(18):2241-2248.

36. Corrado D, Thiene G, Nava A, Rossi L, Pennelli N. Sudden death in young competitive athletes: clinicopathologic correlations in 22 cases. *Am J Med.* 1990;89(5):588-596.
37. Luijkx T, Velthuis BK, Prakken NH, et al. Impact of revised Task Force Criteria: distinguishing the athlete's heart from ARVC/D using cardiac magnetic resonance imaging. *Eur J Prev Cardiol.* 2012;19(4):885-891.
38. Tandri H, Asimaki A, Abraham T, et al. Prolonged RV endocardial activation duration: a novel marker of arrhythmogenic right ventricular dysplasia/cardiomyopathy. *Heart Rhythm.* 2009;6(6):769-775.
39. Hébert JL, Duthoit G, Hidden-Lucet F, et al. Images in cardiovascular medicine. Fortuitous discovery of partial Uhl anomaly in a male adult. *Circulation.* 2010;121(22):e426-e429.
40. Uhl HS. A previously undescribed congenital malformation of the heart: almost total absence of the myocardium of the right ventricle. *Bull Johns Hopkins Hosp.* 1952;91(3):197-209.
41. Hunold P, Wieneke H, Bruder O, et al. Late enhancement: a new feature in MRI of arrhythmogenic right ventricular cardiomyopathy? *J Cardiovasc Magn Reson.* 2005;7(4):649-655.
42. Nava A, Bauce B, Basso C, et al. Clinical profile and long-term follow-up of 37 families with arrhythmogenic right ventricular cardiomyopathy. *J Am Coll Cardiol.* 2000;36(7):2226-2233.
43. Corrado D, Basso C, Thiene G, et al. Spectrum of clinicopathologic manifestations of arrhythmogenic right ventricular cardiomyopathy/dysplasia: a multicenter study. *J Am Coll Cardiol.* 1997;30(6):1512-1520.
44. Paetsch I, Reith S, Gassler N, Jahnke C. Isolated arrhythmogenic left ventricular cardiomyopathy identified by cardiac magnetic resonance imaging. *Eur Heart J.* 2011;32(22):2840.

7

Drug Therapy in Arrhythmogenic Right Ventricular Cardiomyopathy/Dysplasia: When and How to Use Which Drugs

Thomas Wichter, MD

Introduction

Arrhythmogenic right ventricular cardiomyopathy/dysplasia (ARVC/D) is a major cause of sudden death and ventricular tachyarrhythmias in young, apparently healthy individuals and athletes.[1-3] Mutations in genes encoding for desmosomal cell contact proteins result in myocyte death and myocardial atrophy with subsequent fibrofatty replacement, predominantly affecting right ventricular myocardium.[3-5] The left ventricular myocardium may be involved early in the disease process.[6] These pathomorphological alterations result in the major clinical manifestations of ARVC/D:

1. Ventricular tachyarrhythmias due to the arrhythmogenic substrate, mainly with areas of slow conduction and dispersion of refractoriness
2. Heart failure due to global and/or regional right and/or left ventricular dysfunction

Clinical Presentation

ARVC/D usually presents with ventricular tachyarrhythmias of left bundle branch block (LBBB) configuration in apparently healthy adolescents or young adults. In most cases, the age at the time of first manifestation ranges between 15 and 40 years. First symptoms of ARVC/D during early childhood or beyond the age of 60 years are unusual. Men are more frequently affected than women and present with more extensive disease expression.[1,3]

In the majority of patients, ARVC/D manifests first with the sporadic occurrence of monomorphic ventricular tachycardia (VT). Others present with frequent premature ventricular beats, sporadic or repetitive ventricular runs, or nonsustained VT. Associated symptoms range from palpitations and paroxysmal tachycardia to dizziness, syncope, or sudden cardiac arrest. Primary ventricular fibrillation is rare but may occur as a first manifestation in early phases of "concealed" ARVC/D.

Current Concepts in Arrhythmogenic Right Ventricular Cardiomyopathy/Dysplasia

Clinical signs of heart failure are usually limited to patients with advanced right ventricular dysfunction and/or left ventricular involvement, both occurring mostly in later stages of ARVC/D and in patients with a long history of ventricular arrhythmias.

Diagnostic criteria for ARVC/D were proposed and updated by an international study group.[7,8] The catalogue includes morphofunctional, ECG (depolarization and repolarization), arrhythmia, histopathologic, and genetic criteria.

Risk Stratification

The natural history of ARVC/D is mainly affected by the electrical instability of the myocardium, which may lead to ventricular tachyarrhythmias and sudden death at any time during the disease course. The proportion of ARVC/D as the underlying disease in cases of sudden cardiac death is unknown but has been estimated to be 15%–25% in patients below 35 years of age.[9] These data correspond well with the "natural history" of ARVC/D, with mortality rates of up to 25% after 10 years on empiric (uncontrolled) antiarrhythmic drug therapy.[10-14] In advanced stages of ARVC/D, progression of right and/or left ventricular dysfunction may result in right or biventricular heart failure, increasing the risk of cardiac death.[15-18] Therefore, ARVC/D is not a benign disease but requires effective risk stratification and tailored treatment to reduce symptoms and to prevent sudden cardiac death or progressive heart failure.

Various studies identified clinical variables to stratify the risk for life-threatening ventricular tachyarrhythmias or sudden cardiac death in ARVC/D (Table 7.1),[3] helping to separate high-risk patients with an indication for the implantation of a cardioverter-defibrillator (ICD) from intermediate- or low-risk patients in whom antiarrhythmic drug therapy, beta-blockers, or even no treatment may be sufficiently safe and effective.

TABLE 7.1 Risk factors for ventricular tachyarrhythmias and sudden arrhythmic death in ARVC/D

MAJOR RISK FACTORS
• Survived cardiac arrest or ventricular fibrillation (VF) • Sustained VT with hemodynamic compromise (unstable VT) • Unexplained syncope
INTERMEDIATE RISK FACTORS
• Sustained VT without hemodynamic compromise (stable VT) • Nonsustained VT (Holter or exercise tests) • Severe right ventricular dysfunction • Left ventricular involvement or symptomatic heart failure • Early onset of severe structural disease (age ≤ 35 years) • Physical exercise and sports activity
MINOR OR CONTROVERSIAL RISK FACTORS
• Family history of sudden cardiac death (age ≤ 35 years) • "Malignant" genetic mutations (ie, compound heterozygosity, digenic mutations) • Frequent premature ventricular complexes (PVCs) • QRS prolongation, QRS dispersion, or delayed S-wave upstroke in ECG leads V_1–V_2 • Inducibility of VT during programmed ventricular stimulation (PVS) • Electroanatomical scar or fractionated signals on voltage mapping (CARTO®, Biosense Webster, Diamond Bar, CA)

Treatment Targets and Options

In patients with ARVC/D, therapeutic options and modalities include lifestyle advice (ie, discourage from competitive sports), pharmacologic treatment, catheter ablation, ICD implantation, and heart transplantation. Major aims and targets for treatment and clinical management include:

- reduction of mortality (arrhythmic sudden death and death from heart failure)
- reduction of VT recurrences and ICD interventions (appropriate or inappropriate)
- prevention of disease acceleration with progression of arrhythmias and of right and/or left ventricular dysfunction with heart failure

- reduction of symptoms from arrhythmias and/or heart failure
- maintenance or improvement of exercise capacity and quality of life.

Most of the data on treatment and long-term outcome refer to retrospective analyses in single centers with limited numbers of patients. Controlled, randomized trials have not been published, and international registries[19-21] have reported only limited data on drug treatment so far.

It is difficult to compare patient cohorts from different centers because of differences in patient selection (ie, referral bias) and application of diagnostic criteria. In addition, treatment strategies may be different in centers or countries with potential changes and evolution over time. In this context, it is important to realize that algorithms for the treatment of arrhythmias have changed over the past decades with an increase of ICD implantations and decrease in the first-line use of antiarrhythmic drugs and catheter ablation in ventricular arrhythmias in general and in patients with ARVC/D in particular.

Exercise and Sports

ARVC/D is of increasing interest in sports medicine, particularly with regard to sports eligibility, preparticipation screening, and follow-up evaluation of athletes.[22,23] This is because of the increased risk of sudden death due to the propensity for ventricular arrhythmias. In this context, it has been shown that physical exercise increases the risk of sudden death by a factor of 5 in young patients with ARVC/D.[24] In addition, exercise and sports increase the potential for accelerated disease progression due to right ventricular volume overload and mechanical stretch impacting on the myocardium affected by a genetically determined damage of mechanical cell-to-cell adhesion contacts.[5,23-25] Therefore, patients with ARVC should be advised against strenuous exercise and vigorous training and should be disqualified from participation in competitive or professional athletic sports. In healthy gene carriers, however, restriction from sports activity is more controversial.

Preload-Reducing Therapy

In a transgenic animal model of heterozygous plakoglobin-deficient mice, Kirchhof et al[26] demonstrated that endurance training accelerated the development of right ventricular dysfunction and arrhythmias. These findings suggest that chronic volume overload and exercise-induced myocardial stretch might contribute to manifestation and progression of ARVC/D.

Using the same mouse model, the authors provided experimental evidence that pharmacological preload-reducing therapy with nitrates and furosemide prevents or slows the development of training-induced ARVC/D in genetically susceptible hearts.[27,28] Trained plakoglobin-deficient mice protected by load-reducing drug therapy showed no signs of accelerated right ventricular dilatation or arrhythmias (VT inducibility) and were not different in phenotype when compared with their wild-type littermates.

However, the insights from these animal models demonstrating beneficial effects of preload-reducing drug therapy with diuretics and nitrates are not yet part of clinical practice. These insights need to be transferred to the clinical arena in patients with early manifestations of ARVC/D in which protection of disease acceleration requires confirmation. For this purpose, a first controlled, prospective, multicenter clinical trial (PreVENT-ARVC®) will soon be initiated in such patients under the leadership of the University Hospital of Münster, Germany.[28]

Treatment of Heart Failure

The prevalence of symptomatic heart failure resulting from right and/or left ventricular dysfunction varies considerably in different ARVC/D cohorts, mainly depending on selection of patients, application of diagnostic criteria, and reason for referral (arrhythmias vs heart failure).[3] Formerly, left ventricular involvement was considered to occur late during a progressive course of ARVC/D. More recently, it has consistently been demonstrated by pathology, magnetic resonance imaging (MRI), and genotype–phenotype correlations that left ventricular involvement may occur also in early phases of ARVC/D and may even be more dominant than right ventricular dysfunction.[4,29,30]

Despite the presence of right, left, or biventricular dysfunction, symptomatic heart failure requiring dedicated medication develops in only a minority of patients with ARVC/D. Studies from different cohorts report variable proportions of patients medically treated for heart failure, ranging from approximately 10% to 30%.[3]

Drug therapy for heart failure in ARVC/D patients follows general heart failure guidelines. Symptomatic right heart failure is treated with vasodilators, nitrates, and diuretics. Pharmacologic treatment of biventricular heart failure and symptomatic left ventricular dysfunction includes angiotensin-converting enzyme (ACE) inhibitors, beta-blockers, mineralocorticoid receptor antagonists (MRA), and diuretics (in case of fluid retention).

In the very rare situation of end-stage heart failure refractory to optimal medical therapy, heart transplantation may be a final option for treatment of severely symptomatic patients with ARVC/D.[31]

Antithrombotic Therapy

In ARVC/D, thromboembolic complications may result from intracardiac thrombus formation in ventricular aneurysms and sacculations or ventricular dilatation due to global or regional right and/or left ventricular dysfunction. A retrospective study by Wlodarska et al[32] reported an annual incidence of 0.5% in 126 patients with ARVC/D followed for 99 ± 64 months. Long-term oral anticoagulation is generally indicated for secondary prevention in patients with documented intracavitary thrombosis or venous or systemic embolism. However, prophylactic anticoagulation only on the basis of morphological or functional risk factors for thromboembolism is much more controversial and is currently not considered to be indicated.

Role of Beta-Blockers

Particularly in early stages of ARVC/D, ventricular arrhythmias and cardiac arrest frequently occur during or immediately after physical exercise or may be triggered by catecholamines. Autonomic dysfunction with increased adrenergic stimulation of the myocardium and subsequent reduction of β-adrenoceptor density was demonstrated by Wichter et al with the use of radionuclide imaging and quantitative positron emission tomography[33,34] and provided a pathophysiological rationale for these clinical observations.

Therefore, antiadrenergic treatment with beta-blockers alone or as an adjunct therapy has been recommended by many authors to prevent exercise-related catecholaminergic ventricular arrhythmias in ARVC/D. On the other hand, the prophylactic use of beta-blockers to improve arrhythmic prognosis and delay disease progression in asymptomatic ARVC/D patients at low risk and healthy gene carriers is more controversial.

Another important indication for beta-blockers in ARVC/D patients is to provide an antiadrenergic adjunct to antiarrhythmic drug therapy for the prevention, suppression, and treatment of symptomatic ventricular arrhythmias. Moreover, beta-blockers are essential as an adjunct treatment to reduce appropriate ICD interventions (VT burden) and to prevent inappropriate ICD shocks resulting from exercise-induced sinus tachycardia, supraventricular tachycardia, or atrial fibrillation with rapid ventricular conduction.

Antiarrhythmic Drug Therapy

In ARVC/D patients, treatment to improve symptoms and prognosis is mainly directed toward the prevention and management of the clinically dominant problem of ventricular arrhythmias, whereas the treatment of symptomatic heart failure is relevant for only a minority of ARVC/D patients. Antiarrhythmic treatment options in ARVC/D include anti-arrhythmic drugs, catheter ablation, and ICD therapy (Figure 7.1).

Experience with the use of antiarrhythmic drugs in patients with coronary artery disease or cardiomyopathies are not transferable to patients with ARVC/D. Prospective randomized studies to compare antiarrhythmic modalities have not been conducted so far. Therefore, current knowledge and recommendations follow an empiric approach and are based on retrospective analyses, registry data, expert opinion and consensus, and individual decisions. Adding further to the complexity of evaluating antiarrhythmic treatment efficacy during long-term follow-up, recurrent arrhythmic events in ARVC/D patients result in frequent changes of antiarrhythmic drugs and dosages as well as modifications of antiarrhythmic strategies and modalities (drugs, ablation, ICD) to treat and prevent ventricular tachyarrhythmias.

In ARVC/D, antiarrhythmic drug therapy may be used to:

- prevent VT recurrence and arrhythmia worsening as a first-line therapy in patients at low or intermediate risk
- reduce VT burden and ICD discharges as an adjunct therapy to ICD implantation or catheter ablation in patients at intermediate and high risk
- reduce emergency hospital admissions and improve quality of life
- prevent sudden arrhythmic death (questionable and unproven)

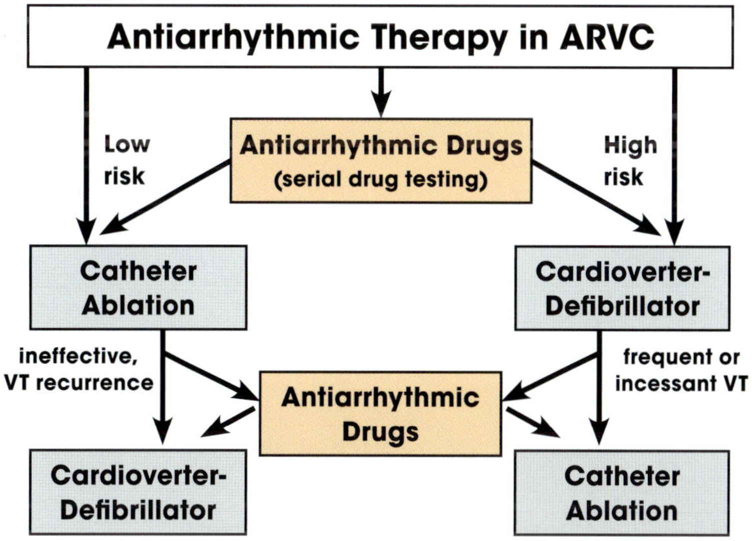

FIGURE 7.1 Stepwise treatment for ventricular tachycardia in patients with ARVC/D. See text for details. *Source:* Adapted from Wichter T, Corrado D, Paul M[35] with kind permission from *Springer Science and Business Media.*

The European Experience (Münster, Germany)

The largest experience on the efficacy of antiarrhythmic drug therapy in ARVC/D comes from Münster (Germany) and was first published by Wichter et al in 1992[36] in a nonrandomized study, which was updated in 2005.[37] The updated series reports on 608 antiarrhythmic drug tests in 191 ARVC/D patients at low or intermediate risk of sudden death. All patients underwent programmed ventricular stimulation in the drug-free state according to a standardized protocol including catecholamine provocation. Patients at high risk of sudden death with a primary indication for ICD implantation were excluded from serial drug testing.

Acute Antiarrhythmic Drug Efficacy. Acute antiarrhythmic drug efficacy was tested for various agents by serial programmed ventricular stimulation in patients with inducible VT ($n = 122$) and by serial noninvasive Holter monitoring and exercise tests in patients without inducible VT during programmed stimulation (noninducible; $n = 69$).

Criteria to evaluate the acute efficacy of antiarrhythmic drug therapy are difficult to define because they may vary with the clinical situation, the arrhythmia characteristics, and the appropriateness of test modalities to assess a treatment effect. To assess the acute efficacy of antiarrhythmic drugs, the following criteria were used in this study:[36]

Complete efficacy of antiarrhythmic drug therapy was defined as total suppression of inducible VT during electrophysiologic study or suppression and control of incessant VT or VT clusters. In noninducible VT, complete efficacy was considered as a $>90\%$ reduction of ventricular ectopy on Holter and exercise tests and no residual nonsustained or sustained VT.

Partial efficacy of antiarrhythmic drug therapy was considered if VT was rendered more difficult to induce during electrophysiologic study or if only nonclinical VT was induced on the drug. In noninducible VT, partial efficacy was defined as a $>70\%$ but $<90\%$ reduction of ventricular ectopy on Holter or exercise tests.

Drug failure was defined as unchanged VT induction during electrophysiologic study, in-hospital VT recurrence, or failure to control incessant or frequent VT recurrences. In noninducible VT, no significant reduction or even an increase of ventricular ectopy on Holter or exercise tests was considered a drug failure.

The updated series by Wichter et al[37] showed that complete antiarrhythmic drug efficacy occurred in 62% of 191 patients and partial efficacy in another 13% of patients, resulting in a total overall acute efficacy rate of 75%. Figure 7.2 depicts the complete, partial, and over-

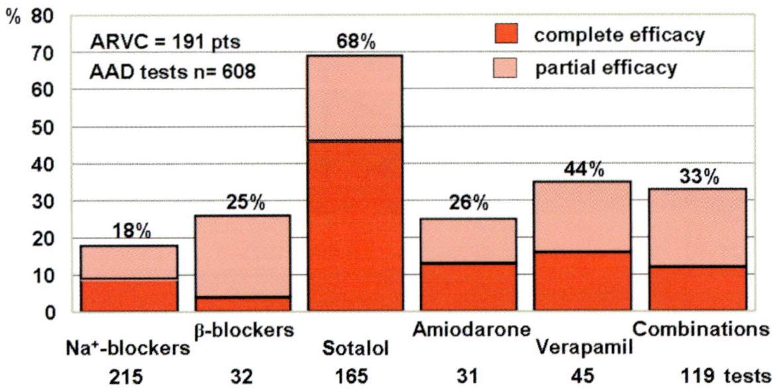

FIGURE 7.2 Efficacy rates of different antiarrhythmic drugs for treatment of VT in ARVC/D ($n = 191$ patients, $n = 608$ tests). See text for details and efficacy criteria. AAD = antiarrhythmic drug. *Source:* Adapted from Wichter T, Borggrefe M, Böcker D, Breithardt G,[38] with kind permission from Wiley-Blackwell, Inc.

all efficacy rates for different antiarrhythmic agents. Multivariate analysis identified extensive right ventricular dysfunction as an independent predictor of antiarrhythmic drug failure.

Sotalol in a relatively high dosage of 320–480 mg/day (releasing its class-III antiarrhythmic potential) was identified as the most effective drug with a 68% overall acute success rate. Of the patients with inducible VT who did not respond to oral sotalol, all but one proved refractory to all other antiarrhythmic agents tested (including amiodarone). Side effects requiring withdrawal of sotalol treatment were rare (5.5%) and mostly occurred within the first days of therapy.[36]

Amiodarone alone was reported with similar or less favorable results when compared with sotalol. Of 12 patients receiving both drugs successively, 1 of 8 sotalol nonresponders was effectively treated with amiodarone, whereas 2 of 9 amiodarone nonresponders were effectively treated with sotalol.[36] The combination of amiodarone with beta-blockers was more effective than amiodarone alone.[37] However, given the high incidence of serious side effects of amiodarone during long-term treatment, amiodarone should not be recommended as a first-line drug in a young patient with ARVC/D. Therefore, sotalol or nonpharmacological treatment options should be considered prior to initiation of long-term amiodarone therapy.

Class-1 antiarrhythmic drugs proved effective in only a minority of patients with ARVC (18%), although some patients received 3 or more different class-1 drugs successively without satisfactory antiarrhythmic efficacy. Class-1c agents appeared to be slightly more effective than class-1a and class-1b drugs.[36,37]

Beta-blockers and verapamil were tested in only a small proportion of ARVC/D patients with noninducible, nonreentrant VT and presumed mechanisms of triggered activity or abnormal automaticity. In this particular subgroup, beta-blockers and verapamil demonstrated overall efficacy rates of 25% and 44%, respectively. However, they were not likely to be successful in reentrant arrhythmias.[37]

Drug combinations of class-1 drugs with amiodarone or sotalol were effective in a minority of patients with ARVC/D in whom the individual drugs had previously failed. Combinations of 2 class-1 drugs and class-1 drugs with beta-blockers were not effective in any of these patients.[37]

Long-Term Antiarrhythmic Drug Efficacy. Long-term antiarrhythmic drug efficacy (mean follow-up, 53 ± 32 months) was assessed in all 143 ARVC/D patients discharged on an antiarrhythmic drug. The incidence of sudden death was low (4 of 143 patients = 2.8%, or 0.6% per year) and the overall rate of nonfatal VT recurrence was acceptable (25% after 5 years). Patients who were discharged on a drug that was tested to be effective had a favorable prognosis. In contrast, in patients with unsuccessful serial drug testing, noncompliant drug intake, or inadequate dosage, the ventricular tachyarrhythmia recurrence rate approached 60% after 3 years[37] (Figure 7.3).

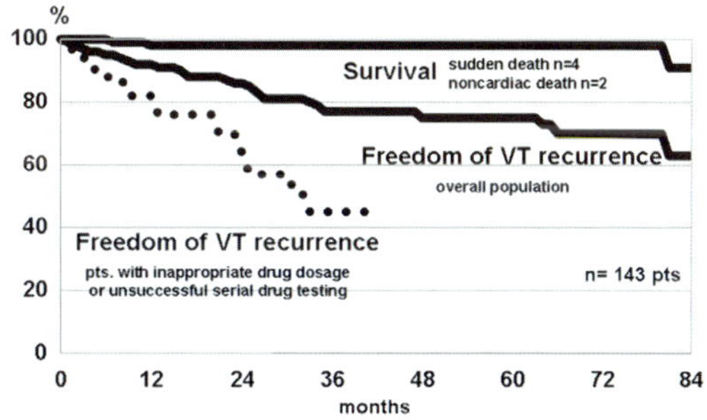

FIGURE 7.3 Long-term outcome (mean follow-up, 53 ± 32 months) of 143 patients with ARVC/D and low or intermediate risk of sudden death discharged on antiarrhythmic drugs after serial drug testing. See text for details. *Source:* Adapted from Wichter T, Paul M, Eckardt L, et al,[37] with kind permission from Springer Science and Business Media.

The North American Experience (Multicenter Study). Marcus et al[39] recently published the results of empiric antiarrhythmic drug therapy in an observational study of 108 patients derived from the Multicenter Study on ARVC/D conducted in North America.[20] The ARVC/D patients enrolled were at high risk of sudden death, reflected by high rates of ICD implantation (88%) and beta-blocking agents (61%) at baseline. Patients were treated with additional antiarrhythmic drugs at the discretion of the treating physician on an empiric basis with no systematic approach to test drug efficacy.

During a mean follow-up period of 16 ± 13 months, 235 ventricular arrhythmic events were observed in 32 patients (30%). Beta-blockers provided no clinical benefit with regard to prevention of VT or ventricular fibrillation when compared with patients not taking beta-blockers or antiarrhythmic drugs. However, there was a trend (not statistically significant) toward a reduction of ICD shocks. Low-dose sotalol with a mean dose of 240 mg per day was administered on an empiric basis in 38 patients. The incidence of clinically relevant ventricular arrhythmias or ICD shocks was not affected; therefore, no arrhythmic protection was observed in patients treated with sotalol. However, the cycle length of recurrent VT was prolonged, resulting in slower heart rate during VT. Only the small subgroup of 10 patients receiving amiodarone showed a reduction of ventricular tachycardia recurrences and appropriate ICD interventions when compared with all other patients in this study. These data, however, should be interpreted with caution because of the small numbers of patients treated and the potential selection bias involved.[39]

Comparison of Major Antiarrhythmic Drug Studies. Discrepancies between the North American study by Marcus et al[39] and the European experience reported by Wichter et al[36,37] mainly relate to the efficacy of antiarrhythmic drugs for the suppression of VT in general and to the efficacy of sotalol in particular. The 2 studies differ with respect to study populations (high-risk patients with an ICD vs low- or intermediate-risk patients), sotalol dosages (160–320 vs 320–480 mg/day), treatment guidance (empiric vs guided by electrophysiological study or Holter and exercise tests), and follow-up duration (16 ± 13 vs 53 ± 32 months).

Other Clinical Studies and Expert Opinions. Other data on antiarrhythmic drug therapy in ARVC/D are weaker and of less clinical importance than those from the 2 major studies discussed above.

The European multicenter ICD study published by Corrado et al[40] reported on 132 patients with ARVC/D and implantable ICDs. In patients with an index episode of hemodynamically unstable VT, syncope, or survived cardiac arrest, the majority of potentially life-saving ICD interventions occurred despite an adjunct empiric antiarrhythmic drug therapy. It was concluded that in high-risk patients with ARVC/D, such empiric antiarrhythmic treatment does not protect against sudden death but may reduce the number of VT episodes (VT burden) and ICD interventions (shock delivery in particular). Of the 132 total study patients, 104 (79%) received antiarrhythmic drugs in addition to the implanted ICD. Sotalol (36%), amiodarone alone (8%) or combined with beta-blockers (13%), beta-blockers alone (20%), and flecainide (2%) were used as antiarrhythmic agents. During follow-up of 39 ± 25 months, 53 of 64 patients (83%) with appropriate ICD therapies (48%) were on an antiarrhythmic drug at the time of the first ICD intervention. Compared with the 51 of 68 patients (75%) with no or inappropriate ICD interventions, there was no difference in antiarrhythmic drug efficacy. The incidence of ventricular flutter or fibrillation as a surrogate for "hypothetical sudden death" did not differ in the groups with and without antiarrhythmic drug therapy, nor was a difference found in incidence of flutter/fibrillation among patients on different antiarrhythmic drugs.[40]

On the other hand, a subgroup analysis from the same study[40] indicated that patients with an index episode of VT without hemodynamic compromise had a favorable long-term course without life-threatening ventricular tachyarrhythmia recurrences (ventricular flutter or fibrillation) requiring ICD interventions. This indicates the potential role for antiarrhythmic drug therapy in the intermediate risk cohort with hemodynamically stable VT as an index event.

The German single-center experience from Münster reported similar results in high-risk patients after ICD implantation[41] and in intermediate- or low-risk patients treated by antiarrhythmic drugs or catheter ablation.[37] Also, the Johns Hopkins experience from Baltimore reported comparable data on ICD therapy and drug treatment in a cohort of ARVC/D patients with implanted defibrillators.[42]

Pezawas et al[43] also confirmed these results and reported a low risk if the clinical index VT or the induced VT was slower and hemodynamically well tolerated. In such patients, a conservative approach with antiarrhythmic drug therapy guided by programmed ventricular stimulation was selected and resulted in good long-term outcomes.

Several small studies confirmed the efficacy of high-dose sotalol and amiodarone with adjunct beta-blockade, both providing similar results in suppressing VT recurrences.[13,14] The combination of amiodarone with beta-blockers may be more effective than the individual drugs alone. Both therapeutic regimens consist of a combination of class-3 antiarrhythmic properties plus beta-blockade, which appears to act synergistically in patients with ARVC/D. This may be due to the strong catecholamine dependence as a triggering factor for ventricular arrhythmia in many of these patients. However, whether these antiarrhythmic drug strategies improve prognosis by the prevention of sudden death remains unproven.

Monitoring of Antiarrhythmic Drug Efficacy. The available data indicate and confirm that adequate monitoring of drug efficacy is a mandatory prerequisite for long-term antiarrhythmic drug therapy in ARVC/D. Empiric antiarrhythmic drug treatment without evidence for appropriate suppression of the clinical arrhythmia cannot be recommended due to a high incidence of VT recurrences and a significant mortality from sudden death during long-term follow-up.[10-14,39] In contrast, the assessment of antiarrhythmic drug efficacy by serial electrophysiologic studies (inducible VT) or Holter monitoring combined with exercise testing and/or provocation with intravenous catecholamines (noninducible VT) provided better long-term outcomes when compared with empiric drug treatment.[36,37,43]

In this context, it is important to stress the role of follow-up visits at regular and scheduled intervals during the long-term course of ARVC/D, not only to detect disease progression, but also to improve and optimize drug therapy and patient compliance. During routine follow-up visits on antiarrhythmic drug therapy, particular attention should be given to arrhythmias and the QRS width (class-1 drugs) and the QT interval (class-3 and class-1a drugs) in 12-lead resting ECG, exercise test, and Holter monitoring. In addition, electrolyte disturbances (especially hypokalemia) should be avoided, and attention should be given to potential drug interactions (particularly those with QT prolongation) in order to prevent proarrhythmic drug effects. Serial echocardiography and/or MRI is useful for the early detection of disease progression and development of right and/or left ventricular dysfunction and heart failure.

Conclusion

The available evidence suggests that healthy gene carriers carry the lowest arrhythmic risk and do not require any treatment. Restriction from sports activity is controversial, and prophylactic therapy with beta-blockers to prevent disease development or occurrence of arrhythmic events is not established in these individuals.

Since physical exercise has been shown to increase the risk of sudden death fivefold in patients with ARVC/D, asymptomatic and symptomatic patients should be recommended to refrain from sports activity. Preload-reducing treatment with nitrates and diuretics showed promising effects to prevent disease progression in a transgenic mouse model, but this requires confirmation in human studies. However, heart failure medication, including ACE inhibitors, mineralocorticoid receptor antagonists (MRA), and beta-blockers, is established in patients with advanced disease and symptomatic, severe right, left, or biventricular dysfunction.

Prophylactic beta-blocker therapy to reduce the rate of arrhythmic complications and ARVC/D progression is controversial. However, beta-blockers should be considered in those individuals with induction or worsening of ventricular arrhythmias with exercise. In addition, they are an important adjunct for the prevention of inappropriate ICD therapies.

Antiarrhythmic therapy is not required in healthy gene carriers and asymptomatic ARVC/D patients without risk factors. However, such individuals should be followed on a regular basis by noninvasive cardiac evaluations for early detection of warning signs and symptoms and for the timely identification of disease progression or ventricular arrhythmias. First-line treatment with antiarrhythmic drugs is indicated in patients with symptomatic, frequent premature ventricular beats, nonsustained VT, or hemodynamically well-tolerated sustained VT. In addition, antiarrhythmic medication is recommended as an adjunct treatment to catheter ablation and/or ICD therapy to reduce VT burden and ICD discharges. The available evidence suggests that antiarrhythmic drug therapy with either sotalol or amiodarone in combination with beta-blockers provides best results, with equal efficacy and a relatively low proarrhythmic risk. However, their ability to prevent sudden cardiac death is unproven.

In patients with ARVC/D and survived cardiac arrest, hemodynamically unstable VT, or unexplained syncope (secondary prevention), or in those at high risk of such life-threatening events (primary prevention), the implantation of an ICD is indicated and provides safe and effective termination of malignant ventricular tachyarrhythmias.[40,41,44-46] However, this is at the cost of a relevant incidence of inappropriate ICD discharges (due to supraventricular arrhythmias or oversensing) and lead-related complications during the long-term course after ICD implantation.[41,45] Therefore, risk-adapted and tailored treatment algorithms are warranted for the management of ventricular arrhythmias in ARVC/D.[3,35,44]

Abbreviations

ICD	implantable cardioverter-defibrillator
LBBB	left bundle branch block
PVC	premature ventricular contraction
VF	ventricular fibrillation
VT	ventricular tachycardia

References

1. Marcus FI, Fontaine G, Guiraudon G, et al. Right ventricular dysplasia: a report of 24 cases. *Circulation*. 1982;65:384-399.
2. Thiene G, Nava A, Corrado D, Rossi L, Pennelli N. Right ventricular cardiomyopathy and

sudden cardiac death in young people. *N Eng J Med.* 1988;318:129-133.
3. Basso C, Corrado D, Bauce B, Thiene G. Arrhythmogenic right ventricular cardiomyopathy. *Circ Arrhythm Electrophysiol.* 2012;5:1233-1246.
4. Corrado D, Basso C, Pilichou K, Thiene G. Molecular biology and clinical management of arrhythmogenic right ventricular cardiomyopathy/dysplasia. *Heart.* 2011;97:530-539.
5. Marcus FI, Edson S, Towbin JA. Genetics of arrhythmogenic right ventricular cardiomyopathy: a practical guide for physicians. *J Am Coll Cardiol.* 2013;61:1945-1948.
6. Corrado D, Basso C, Thiene G, et al. Spectrum of clinicopathologic manifestations of arrhythmogenic right ventricular cardiomyopathy/dysplasia: a multicenter study. *J Am Coll Cardiol.* 1997;30:1512-1520.
7. McKenna WJ, Thiene G, Nava A, et al. Diagnosis of arrhythmogenic right ventricular dysplasia/cardiomyopathy. Task Force of the Working Group Myocardial and Pericardial Disease of the European Society of Cardiology and of the Scientific Council on Cardiomyopathies of the International Society and Federation of Cardiology. *Br Heart J.* 1994;71:215-218.
8. Marcus FI, McKenna WJ, Sherrill D, et al. Diagnosis of arrhythmogenic right ventricular cardiomyopathy/dysplasia: proposed modification of the Task Force Criteria. *Eur Heart J.* 2010;31:806-814.
9. Corrado D, Basso C, Thiene G. Pathological findings in victims of sport-related sudden cardiac death. *Sports Exerc Injury.* 1996;2:78-86.
10. Blomström-Lundqvist C, Sabel KG, Olsson SB. A long-term follow up of 15 patients with arrhythmogenic right ventricular dysplasia. *Br Heart J.* 1987;58:477-488.
11. Marcus FI, Fontaine GH, Frank R, Gallagher JJ, Reiter MJ. Long-term follow-up in patients with arrhythmogenic right ventricular disease. *Eur Heart J.* 1989;10(Suppl. D):68-73.
12. Canu G, Atallah G, Claudel JP, et al. Prognostic et évolution à long terme de la dysplasie arythmogène du ventricule droit. *Arch Mal Cœur Vaiss.* 1993;86:41-48.
13. Leclercq JF, Coumel P, Denjoy I, et al. Long-term follow-up after sustained monomorphic ventricular tachycardia: causes, pump failure, and empiric antiarrhythmic therapy that modify survival. *Am Heart J.* 1991;121:1685-1692.
14. Naccarella F, Naccarelli G, Fattori R, et al. Arrhythmogenic right ventricular dysplasia: cardiomyopathy current opinions on diagnostic and therapeutic aspects. *Curr Opin Cardiol.* 2001;16:8-16.
15. Hulot S, Jouven X, Empana JP, Frank R, Fontaine G. Natural history and risk stratification of arrhythmogenic right ventricular dysplasia/cardiomyopathy. *Circulation.* 2004;110:1879-1884.
16. Lemola K, Brunckhorst C, Helfenstein U, Oechslin E, Jenni R, Duru F. Predictors of adverse outcome in patients with arrhythmogenic right ventricular dysplasia/cardiomyopathy: long term experience of a tertiary care centre. *Heart.* 2005;91:1167-1172.
17. Kiès P, Bootsma M, Bax J, Schalij MJ, van der Wall EE. Arrhythmogenic right ventricular dysplasia/cardiomyopathy: screening, diagnosis, and treatment. *Heart Rhythm.* 2006;3:225-234.
18. Schuler PK, Haegeli LM, Saguner AM, et al. Predictors of appropriate ICD therapy in patients with arrhythmogenic right ventricular cardiomyopathy: long term experience of a tertiary care center. *PLoS ONE.* 2012;7(9):e39584. doi:10.1371/journal.pone.0039584.
19. Basso C, Wichter T, Danieli GA, et al. Arrhythmogenic right ventricular cardiomyopathy: clinical registry and database, evaluation of therapies, pathology registry, DNA banking. *Eur Heart J.* 2004;25:531-534.
20. Marcus F, Towbin JA, Zareba W, et al. ARVD/C Investigators. Arrhythmogenic right ventricular dysplasia/cardiomyopathy (ARVD/C): a multidisciplinary study–design and protocol. *Circulation.* 2003;107:2975-2978.
21. Marcus FI, Zareba W, Calkins H, et al. Arrhythmogenic right ventricular cardiomyopathy/dysplasia clinical presentation and diagnostic evaluation: results from the North American Multidisciplinary Study. *Heart Rhythm.* 2009;6:984-992.

22. Corrado D, Basso C, Pavei A, Michieli P, Schiavon M, Thiene G. Trends in sudden cardiovascular death in young competitive athletes after implementation of a preparticipation screening program. *JAMA*. 2006;296:1593-1601.
23. Wichter T, Paul M, Breithardt G. Arrhythmogene rechtsventrikuläre Kardiomyopathie: Sportmedizinische Aspekte. *Deutsche Zeitschrift für Sportmedizin*. 2005;56:118-125.
24. Corrado D, Basso C, Rizzoli G, Schiavon M, Thiene G. Does sports activity enhance the risk of sudden death in adolescents and young adults? *J Am Coll Cardiol*. 2003;42:1959-1963.
25. Gerull B, Heuser A, Wichter T, et al. Mutations in the desmosomal arm repeat protein plakophilin-2 are common in arrhythmogenic right ventricular cardiomyopathy. *Nat Genet*. 2004;36:1162-1164.
26. Kirchhof P, Fabritz L, Zwiener M, et al. Age- and training-dependent development of arrhythmogenic right ventricular cardiomyopathy in heterozygous plakoglobin-deficient mice. *Circulation*. 2006;114:1799-1806.
27. Fabritz L, Hoogendijk MG, Scicluna BP, et al. Load-reducing therapy prevents development of arrhythmogenic right ventricular cardiomyopathy in plakoglobin-deficient mice. *J Am Coll Cardiol*. 2011;57:740-750.
28. Fabritz L, Fortmüller L, Yu TY, Paul M, Kirchhof P. Can preload-reducing therapy prevent disease progression in arrhythmogenic right ventricular cardiomyopathy? Experimental evidence and concept for a clinical trial. *Prog Biophys Mol Biol*. 2012;110:340-346.
29. Bauce B, Basso C, Rampazzo A, et al. Clinical profile of four families with arrhythmogenic right ventricular cardiomyopathy caused by dominant desmoplakin mutations. *Eur Heart J*. 2005;26:1666-1675.
30. Sen-Chowdhry S, Prasad SK, Syrris P, et al. Cardiovascular magnetic resonance in arrhythmogenic right ventricular cardiomyopathy revisited: comparison with task force criteria and genotype. *J Am Coll Cardiol*. 2006;48:2132-2140.
31. Tedford RJ, James C, Judge DP, et al. Cardiac transplantation in arrhythmogenic right ventricular dysplasia/cardiomyopathy. *J Am Coll Cardiol*. 2012;59:289-290.
32. Wlodarska EK, Wozniak O, Konka M, Rydlewska-Sadowska W, Biederman A, Hoffman P. Thromboembolic complications in patients with arrhythmogenic right ventricular dysplasia/cardiomyopathy. *Europace*. 2006;8:596-600.
33. Wichter T, Hindricks G, Lerch H, et al. Regional myocardial sympathetic dysinnervation in arrhythmogenic right ventricular cardiomyopathy: an analysis using ^{123}I-Meta-Iodobenzylguanidine scintigraphy. *Circulation*. 1994;89:667-683.
34. Wichter T, Schäfers M, Rhodes CG, et al. Abnormalities of cardiac sympathetic innervation in arrhythmogenic right ventricular cardiomyopathy: quantitative assessment of presynaptic norepinephrine reuptake and postsynaptic beta-adrenergic receptor density with positron emission tomography. *Circulation*. 2000;101:1552-1558.
35. Wichter T, Corrado D, Paul M. Risk stratification and antiarrhythmic drug therapy in arrhythmogenic right ventricular cardiomyopathy/dysplasia (ARVC/D). In: Marcus FI, Nava A, Thiene G (eds.): *Arrhythmogenic RV Cardiomyopathy/Dysplasia*. Milan, Italy: Springer Verlag; 2007:171-180.
36. Wichter T, Borggrefe M, Haverkamp W, Chen X, Breithardt G. Efficacy of antiarrhythmic drugs in patients with arrhythmogenic right ventricular disease. Results in patients with inducible and noninducible ventricular tachycardia. *Circulation*. 1992;86:29-37.
37. Wichter T, Paul M, Eckardt L, et al. Arrhythmogenic right ventricular cardiomyopathy: antiarrhythmic drugs, catheter ablation, or ICD. *Herz*. 2005;30:91-101.
38. Wichter T, Borggrefe M, Böcker D, Breithardt G. What therapies to prevent sudden cardiac death in arrhythmogenic right ventricular cardiomyopathy? In: Aliot E, Clémenty J, Prystowsky EN (eds.): *Fighting Sudden Cardiac Death: A Worldwide Challenge*. Armonk, NY: Futura Publishing; 2000:275-298.

39. Marcus GM, Glidden DV, Polonsky B, et al. Efficacy of antiarrhythmic drugs in arrhythmogenic right ventricular cardiomyopathy. *J Am Coll Cardiol.* 2009;54:609-615.
40. Corrado D, Leoni L, Link MS, et al. Implantable cardioverter-defibrillator therapy for prevention of sudden death in patients with arrhythmogenic right ventricular cardiomyopathy/dysplasia. *Circulation.* 2003;108: 3084-3091.
41. Wichter T, Paul M, Wollmann C, et al. Implantable cardioverter/defibrillator therapy in arrhythmogenic right ventricular cardiomyopathy: single-center experience of long-term follow-up and complications in 60 patients. *Circulation.* 2004;109:1503-1508.
42. Roguin A, Bomma CS, Nasir K, et al. Implantable cardioverter-defibrillators in patients with arrhythmogenic right ventricular dysplasia/cardiomyopathy. *J Am Coll Cardiol.* 2004;43:1843-1852.
43. Pezawas T, Stix G, Kastner J, Schneider B, Wolzt M, Schmidinger H. Ventricular tachycardia in arrhythmogenic right ventricular dysplasia/cardiomyopathy: clinical presentation, risk stratification and results of long-term follow-up. *Int J Cardiol.* 2006;107:360-368.
44. Buja G, Estes NA III, Wichter T, Corrado D, Marcus F, Thiene G. Arrhythmogenic right ventricular cardiomyopathy/dysplasia: risk stratification and therapy. *Prog Cardiovasc Dis.* 2008;50:282-293.
45. Corrado D, Calkins H, Link MS, et al. Prophylactic implantable defibrillator in patients with arrhythmogenic right ventricular cardiomyopathy/dysplasia and no prior ventricular fibrillation or sustained ventricular tachycardia. *Circulation.* 2010;122: 1144-1152.
46. Schinkel AFL. Implantable cardioverter defibrillators in arrhythmogenic right ventricular dysplasia/cardiomyopathy: patient outcomes, incidence of appropriate and inappropriate interventions, and complications. *Circ Arrhythm Electrophysiol.* 2003;6:562-568.

8

The Role of Implantable Defibrillators and Catheter Ablation in the Management of Patients with Arrhythmogenic Right Ventricular Cardiomyopathy/Dysplasia

Florence Porterfield and Hugh Calkins, MD

Introduction

Arrhythmogenic right ventricular cardiomyopathy/dysplasia (ARVC/D) is an inherited cardiomyopathy that is characterized by ventricular arrhythmias, an increased risk of sudden death, and abnormalities of right ventricular structure and function.[1-4] Although structural involvement of the right ventricle predominates, a left ventricular–dominant form of ARVC/D has been described.[5,6] The pathologic hallmark of ARVC/D is myocyte loss with fibrofatty replacement. Since the first detailed clinical description of the disorder in 1982,[1] significant advances have been made in our understanding of all aspects of this disease. Over the last decade, mutations in most desmosomal proteins and also some nondesmosomal proteins have been identified as the genetic basis of ARVC/D. Because a pathogenic mutation can be identified in more than 50% of affected individuals, genetic testing has emerged as an important diagnostic tool.[7,8] The purpose of this chapter is to provide a concise and up-to-date review of the role of catheter ablation and device therapy in the management of ARVC/D.

Implantable Cardioverter-Defibrillator (ICD) Therapy in ARVC/D

Overview

Prevention of sudden cardiac death (SCD) from ventricular arrhythmias is the primary goal of ARVC/D management. If not properly managed, ARVC/D can ultimately lead to SCD in young individuals.[3] Implantable cardioverter-defibrillators (ICDs) are an important treatment strategy for ARVC/D patients. ICD therapy is commonly recommended in conjunction with other strategies, medications, and procedures directed at reducing the frequency of ventricular arrhythmias, including exercise restriction, beta-blockers, antiarrhythmic drug therapy, and catheter ablation.

Although ICD therapy plays an important role in reducing SCD risk, it is important to recognize that device therapy is not without limitations. Treatment with ICDs, especially in young individuals, can have both physical and psychological consequences.[9] The psychological stress brought on by the realities of lifelong ICD therapy, including painful shocks and multiple invasive procedures, should not be underestimated. We advise that psychological support and preoperative assessment be easily accessible to young patients treated with ICDs. In addition, the procedural complications associated with ICD implants can include hemorrhage, device infection, pocket perforation, and lead malfunction.[10]

ICD Therapy

A large number of studies have been performed examining the safety and efficacy of ICD therapy when used in the treatment of patients with ARVC/D.[11-16] These studies, taken as a whole, have demonstrated that patients with ARVC/D who undergo ICD implantation have a high likelihood of receiving an appropriate ICD therapy for treatment of sustained ventricular arrhythmias.

The Johns Hopkins Experience

Over the past 10 years, we have published a number of studies[17-20] that have examined the outcomes of ARVC/D patients who undergo ICD implantation. In performing these studies, we hoped to address the important question of how best to risk stratify patients with ARVC/D. One of our first studies[17] was published in 2004. In this study, we examined the effectiveness of ICD therapy in 42 patients diagnosed with ARVC/D. Thirty-eight (90%) patients received an ICD for primary prevention of SCD. The devices were third- or fourth-generation defibrillators with the capability of storing electrocardiographic data. Twenty-seven (64%) patients received a single-chamber device, and 15 (36%) patients were given a dual-chamber device. The results after the follow-up period of 42 ± 26 months showed that 33 (78%) patients experienced approximately 4 appropriate ICD interventions. Ten (24%) patients had inappropriate interventions, and 5 (12%) patients endured ICD firing storms due to physical exertion. Of the overall cohort, 5 (8%) experienced a complication. Of these, 3 (60%) required lead repositioning attributable to inadequate R-wave amplitude, 1 (20%) underwent system removal and replacement because of an acute infection, and 1 (20%) had a subacute device infection, which was successfully treated with antibiotics. There were no incidences of myocardial perforation or tamponade.

We subsequently performed a study examining the role of electrophysiologic (EP) testing in predicting appropriate ICD therapies in patients with ARVC/D.[18] In this study, particular attention was focused on whether the ICD was implanted for primary or secondary prevention. We enrolled 67 patients (mean age of 36 ± 14 years) with definite or probable ARVC/D who underwent ICD implantation. Appropriate ICD therapies were recorded, and Kaplan-Meier analysis was used to compare the event-free survival time between patients based on the indication for ICD implantation (primary vs secondary prevention), results of EP testing, and whether the patient had probable or definite ARVC/D. Over a mean follow-up of 4.4 ± 2.9 years, 40 of 55 (73%) patients with definite ARVC/D and 4 of 12 (33%) with probable ARVC/D had appropriate ICD therapies for ventricular tachycardia (VT) or ventricular fibrillation (VF) (P = 0.027).[8] Mean time to ICD therapy was 1.1 ± 1.4 years. Eleven of 28 patients (39%) who received an ICD for primary prevention, and 33 of 35 patients (85%) who received an ICD for secondary prevention, experienced appropriate ICD therapies (P = 0.001). EP testing did not predict appropriate ICD interventions in those who received an ICD for primary prevention. Fourteen patients (21%) received ICD therapy for life-threatening (VT/VF > 240 bpm) arrhythmias. There was no difference in the incidence of life-threatening arrhythmias in the primary and secondary prevention groups (P = 0.29). The results of this study revealed that patients who meet the 2010 Task Force Criteria for ARVC/D[8] are at high risk for SCD and should undergo ICD implantation for primary and secondary prevention, regardless of EP testing results.

A more recent study[19] focused on the important issue of the role of ICDs for primary prevention. This study reported the outcomes of 84 patients enrolled in the Johns Hopkins ARVC/D registry who had an ICD implanted for primary prevention of VT or VF. Seventy (83%) patients were diagnosed with definite ARVC/D and 14 (17%) were diagnosed with probable ARVC/D based on the 2010 Task Force Criteria.[8] Thirty (36%) patients had familial ARVC/D, whereas 54 (64%) patients were probands with no family history of the disease. The pathogenic desmosomal mutation was discovered in 36 (43%) individuals after genetic testing. Seventy-two (86%) patients had inducible sustained VT/VF (VT or VF lasting > 30 seconds or that needed to be stopped due to the development of hemodynamic compromise) in a controlled EP study prior to the ICD intervention. The induced VT/VF had a mean cycle length of 257 ± 54 ms. After Holter monitoring in 65 patients, 39 (60%) were determined to have > 1,000 premature ventricular complexes (PVCs)/24 hours. Over a mean follow-up of 4.7 ± 3.4 years, appropriate ICD therapy was seen in 40 (48%) patients, of which 16 (19%) received interventions for rapid VT/VF. Proband status ($P < 0.001$), inducibility at EP study (P = 0.005), presence of nonsustained ventricular tachycardia (NSVT) ($P < 0.001$), and Holter PVC count > 1,000/24 hours (P = 0.024) were identified as significant predictors of appropriate ICD therapy. The 5-year survival free from appropriate ICD therapy for patients with 1, 2, 3, and 4 risk factors was 100%, 83%, 21%, and 15%, respectively. Inducibility at EP study (HR 4.5, 95% CI 1.4–15, P = 0.013) and NSVT (HR 10.5, 95% CI 2.4–46.2, P = 0.002) remained as significant predictors on multivariable analysis. These findings are important as they demonstrate that nearly half of the ARVC/D patients treated with an ICD for primary prevention experienced appropriate ICD interventions. Inducibility at EP study and NSVT are both independent, strong predictors of appropriate ICD therapy. In addition, ventricular ectopy is associated with progressively more common ICD therapy. Incremental risk of ventricular arrhythmias and ICD therapy was observed in the presence of multiple risk factors. In considering these results, it is important to recognize that the use of appropriate ICD therapy due to rapid VT/VF as a surrogate for SCD results in an overestimation of this endpoint.

Our most recent study[20] explored the relationship between phenotypic characteristics and the proposed risk prediction of sustained ventricular arrhythmias in 215 patients with a desmosomal mutation identified through our Johns Hopkins ARVC/D registry. Clinical, electrocardiographic (ECG), and arrhythmic outcome (composite measure of first occurrence of sustained VT/resuscitated SCD/SCD/appropriate ICD therapy) data was obtained for 215 patients (104 families; 85% with pathogenic *PKP-2* mutations). Over a mean follow-up of 7 years, 86 (40%) patients experienced the arrhythmic outcome. Event-free survival was significantly lower among probands ($P < 0.001$) and symptomatic ($P < 0.001$) patients. Integration of ECG repolarization and depolarization abnormalities allowed for differential risk categorization.

Event-free survival at 5 years for the low-risk ECG group (0–1 T inversions or minor depolarization changes) was 97% versus 81% for the intermediate-risk ECG group (2 T inversions + minor depolarization changes) versus 33% for the high-risk ECG group (≥ 3 T inversions ± major or minor depolarization changes) ($P < 0.001$). Incremental arrhythmic risk was seen in patients with increasing PVCs on a Holter ($P < 0.001$). Proband status (HR 7.7; 95% CI 2.8–22.5; $P < 0.001$), ≥ 3 T-wave inversions (HR 4.2; 95% CI 1.2–14.5; $P = 0.035$), and male gender (HR 1.8; 95% CI 1.2–2.8; $P = 0.004$) were independent predictors of the first arrhythmic event on multivariable analysis. Overall, the results of this study revealed that pedigree evaluation, an ECG, and a Holter examination provide for comprehensive arrhythmic risk stratification in patients with ARVC/D associated mutations. Shown in Figure 8.1 is the risk-stratification scheme we developed based on these variables.[20]

As shown in Figure 8.1,[20] the high-risk group (≥ 50%) was composed of (1) probands with high-risk ECG; (2) probands with an intermediate-risk ECG and PVC count > 760/24 hours on a Holter monitor; or (3) family members with a high-risk ECG and PVC count > 760/24 hours on a Holter monitor. The intermediate-risk group (15%–50%) included (1) probands with low-risk ECG; (2) family members with high-risk ECG and PVC count between 11 and 760 on a Holter monitor; and (3) probands with intermediate-risk ECG and PVC count < 760 on a Holter monitor. The low-risk group (< 15%) was made up of (1) family members with a high-risk ECG and < 10 PVC on a Holter monitor and (2) family members with

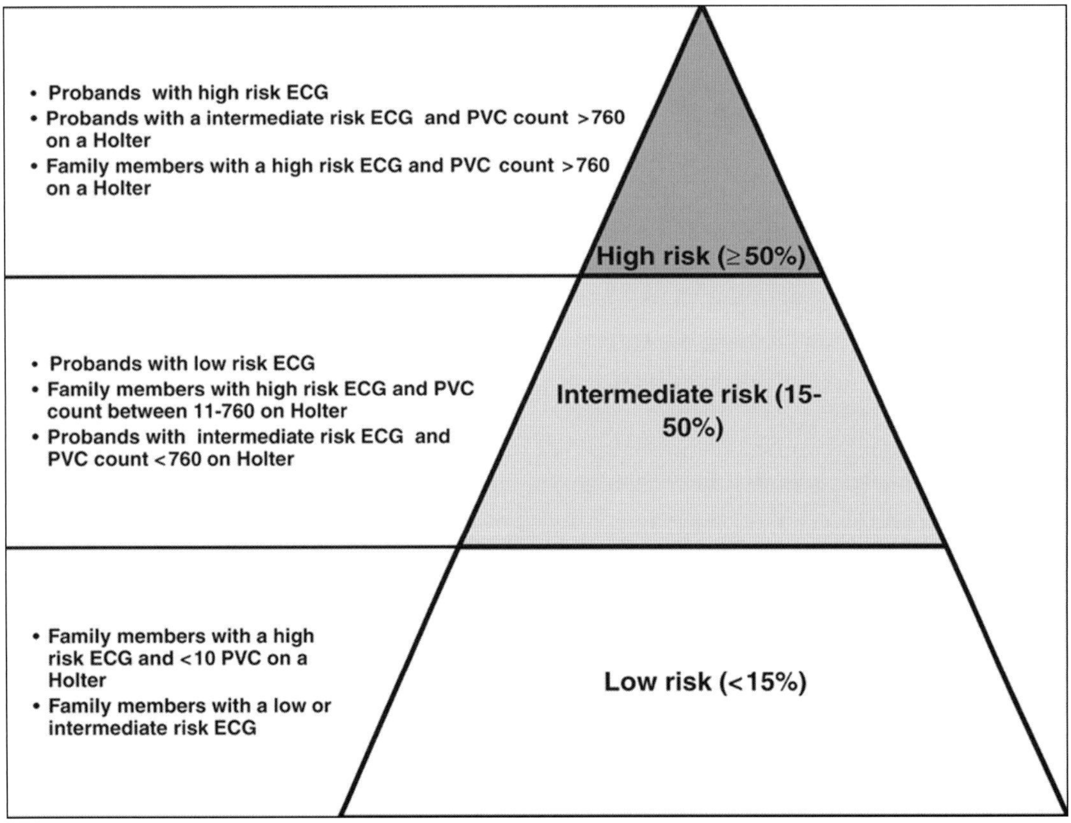

FIGURE 8.1 Proposed risk-prediction scheme based on pedigree, ECG risk categories, and ventricular ectopy. *Source:* Bhonsale A et al.[20]

a low- or intermediate-risk ECG. Our scheme is the first attempt to standardize the risk level of fatal arrhythmias for individuals with the most common ARVC/D gene mutation. Even more important is the fact that these risk stratifications are determined by fundamental clinical tests that can be easily performed. By establishing concrete guidelines, we are helping ARVC/D patients to make the appropriate choice on ICD implantation for the primary prevention of SCD.

Current Indications for ICD Implantation in Patients with ARVC/D

According to the ACC/AHA/HRS 2008 Guidelines for Device-Based Therapy of Cardiac Rhythm Abnormalities,[21] ICD implantation is indicated in patients with structural heart disease who have experienced a sustained ventricular arrhythmia (secondary prevention, Class I indication). These guidelines also state that ICD implantation is reasonable in ARVC/D patients who have one or more risk factors for SCD (IIA indication, level of evidence C).

We are supportive of these recommendations but have applied them with a slightly different perspective. We recommend ICD implantation for all ARVC/D patients who have experienced a sustained ventricular arrhythmia (secondary prevention). We also carefully consider ICD implantation for primary prevention in probands who meet the 2010 Task Force Criteria for ARVC/D.[8] To meet the diagnosis of definite ARVC/D using these diagnostic criteria requires (1) the presence of any 2 of the major criteria; (2) the presence of any combination of 1 major and 2 minor criteria; or (3) the presence of 4 minor criteria.

When discussing the risks and benefits of ICD implantation in this subgroup of patients, we carefully consider whether a particular patient (1) demonstrates the presence or absence of high-risk features such as frequent PVCs, NSVT, cardiac syncope, and severe structural heart disease; (2) whether the patient is willing to give up competitive athletics (ie, participation on a competitive sports team or participation in competitive individual events like marathon running); and (3) the patient's values and preferences. We use a higher threshold for ICD implantation in family members. This reflects the fact that our studies have consistently revealed that family members are at lower risk of experiencing a sustained arrhythmia, are diagnosed earlier in the course of the disease, and, once diagnosed, are encouraged to give up competitive athletics.

Catheter Ablation in ARVC/D

Introduction

Catheter ablation plays an important role in the management of ARVC/D patients who have experienced recurrent symptomatic episodes of sustained VT. It is important to recognize that, unlike patients with idiopathic VT, in which catheter ablation is curative, the role of catheter ablation in patients with ARVC/D is to improve quality of life by decreasing the frequency of episodes of sustained VT, symptomatic NSVT, and frequent ventricular ectopy. Our standard approach is to consider catheter ablation following a trial of beta-blocker therapy and antiarrhythmic therapy (often sotalol or amiodarone). In selected patients who prefer not to be treated with long-term antiarrhythmic drug therapy, we may consider catheter ablation as first-line therapy after a careful discussion of the risks and benefits of catheter ablation versus pharmacologic therapy. Many patients elect to pursue catheter ablation prior to a trial of amiodarone.

History of the Procedure

Catheter ablation was first introduced as a treatment method for drug-resistant VT in the 1980s. The direct-current ablation procedure, termed *fulguration,* utilizes direct current from a defibrillator to shock sites of myocardium that are responsible for the abnormal ventricular activation.[22] Delivered through a catheter, the electric voltage is directly applied to the origins of VT that are identified by endocardial mapping. This aggressive ablative technique, however, is associated with a significant risk of major complications and never gained widespread acceptance.[22,23]

In a pioneering study completed by Fontaine et al,[22] direct-current catheter ablation was evaluated as a therapeutic approach to VT in patients with ARVC/D. The study followed 15 patients with ARVC/D who had undergone fulguration for continuous and drug-resistant VT. Direct-current shocks (160–240 J) were delivered to the endocardial sites of VT origin. Each patient received a series of 1 to 9 shocks during the procedure, except 1 case that was treated with 17 shocks. The results of the patients' 3-month follow-up showed that 6 patients (40%) did not experience recurring VT as a result of one or more fulguration procedures. With the assistance of antiarrhythmic drug therapy, 5 more patients (33%) did not experience a recurrence of VT after one or more fulguration procedures. The study established that direct-current catheter ablation is moderately effective controlling VT in ARVC/D patients, but it also concluded that the procedure has major limitations. To be considered successful in patients with ARVC/D, fulguration requires several high-voltage shocks, multiple sessions, and additional antiarrhythmic drug therapy. In addition, the potential risks associated with utilizing a high-voltage electric current prevent this procedure from being used as first-line treatment of VT in patients with ARVC/D.

Substrate-Based Approach for Radiofrequency Ablation

Radiofrequency (RF) catheter ablation quickly replaced direct-current catheter ablation as the standard ablative technique because it greatly reduced the risks and complications that are associated with direct-current shocks.[22,23] Although the initial approach to RF ablation in patients with ARVC/D involved extensive mapping to identify critical slow zones of conduction during induced VT,[24] this approach has subsequently been replaced by a substrate-based approach. This reflects the fact that precise mapping during VT is challenging in patients with ARVC/D because their VTs are often hemodynamically unstable and also have multiple morphologies. The substrate-based approach involves identification of the exit site of VT using pacemapping followed by ablation of all areas of fractionated electrograms near this exit site.[25] This substrate-based approach is now employed for both endocardial and epicardial ablation procedures in patients with ARVC/D. The substrate-based approach has facilitated the performance of VT ablation procedures in patients previously felt to have "unmappable" VT.[25-28]

In a study completed by Satomi et al,[25] the combined use of conventional mapping as well as a substrate-based approach, with the goal of elimination of all fractionated signals near the exit site of the VT, resulted in ablation success in 23 of 26 (88%) VTs with 26 ± 15 months follow-up. Verma et al[27] further proved the value of substrate-mapping catheter ablation in their study of 22 ARVC/D patients with various other complications including multiple morphologies, NSVT, and hemodynamic intolerance. Each patient underwent detailed electronantomic voltage mapping of the endocardium during sinus rhythm ($n = 21$) or atrially paced rhythm ($n = 1$). Regions with a bipolar electrogram amplitude of < 0.5 mV, 0.5–1.5 mV, and > 1.5 mV were respectively classified as "dense scar," "abnormal," and "normal" myocardium. As a result, areas of scar could be identified in all patients. Based on the detailed maps developed by the 3D CARTO catheter navigation system, linear ablation techniques were used either to encircle the scar or abnormal region or to connect the scar or abnormal tissues to other scar or valve continuity. The results of the substrate-mapping ablative procedure showed success in 18 (82%) patients. During the first, second, and third years of follow-up, VT recurred in 23%, 27%, and 47% of patients, respectively. Both of these studies prove that substrate-based catheter ablation can be successful at controlling VT, especially in patients with complicated forms of ARVC/D.

The Johns Hopkins Experience with VT Ablation in Patients with ARVC/D

Although many studies have reported the safety and efficacy of RF catheter ablation of VT in patients with ARVC/D, we will focus our review on the studies that have been published based on data obtained from the Johns Hopkins ARVC/D registry, which tracks the outcomes of hundreds of patients with ARVC/D across the United States. Our first study,[29] which examined the outcomes of VT ablation in patients with ARVC/D, was published in 2007. In this study, we reported the outcomes of 48 ablation procedures performed in 24 patients with ARVC/D. In particular, we explored the long-term success rates of RF catheter ablation in 24 ARVC/D patients. These 24 patients underwent 48 RF ablation procedures using 4 mm tipped deflectable catheters at 29 different electrophysiology centers in the United States. The results of our study revealed that 46% of procedures were acutely successful and 31% were partially successful (defined as elimination of the clinical VT but persistent inducibility of a nonclinical VT). Twenty-three percent of the RF ablations were acute failures with persistent inducibility of the clinical VT. The cumulative VT-free survival was 75% at 1.5 months, 50% at 5 months, and 25% at 14 months. Surprisingly, the acute success of the procedure did not predict the likelihood of VT recurrence. In 40 (85%) of the procedures, patients experienced VT recurrence at an average of 8 ± 10 months after the procedure. In total, the incidence of VT was 64%, 75%, and 91% at 1, 2, and 3 years, respectively, after a single procedure.

We more recently reported on the outcomes of a larger series of patients with ARVC/D who underwent an endocardial or epicardial VT ablation procedure. In this recent study,[30] we report the outcomes of 87 patients. Twenty-three patients, 19 of whom had experienced at least 1 previously failed endocardial catheter ablation, completed 26 epicardial catheter ablations. Ten of those procedures were solely epicardial ablations, whereas 16 were both epicardial and endocardial procedures. Over a mean follow-up of 88 ± 66 months, the overall freedom from VT was 47%, 21%, and 15% at 1, 5, and 10 years, respectively. The cumulative freedom from VT following epicardial VT ablation was 64% at 1 year and 45% at 5 years. Importantly, the burden of VT decreased following ablation from a median of 0.16 VT episodes per month preablation to 0.08 episodes per month postablation. The results of this study were significant as they demonstrated for the first time that VT ablation reduces the frequency of VT episodes in ARVC/D and also showed that outcomes are improved when an epicardial approach is employed.

Our most recent report[31] focused on the value of catecholamine infusions in triggering VT in patients with ARVC/D. In this study, we looked at the relationship between the morphology of ventricular ectopy and the morphology of induced, sustained VT in 16

ARVC/D patients. The mean baseline PVC frequency was 7,275 (range, 1,353–19,084) per 24 hours. Our approach involved performing a diagnostic EP study at baseline both prior to and following a very high-dose (30 mcg/kg/min) infusion of isoproterenol (Figure 8.2). We recorded 12-lead ECG morphologies of all baseline PVCs preferably at baseline and during a high-dose isoproterenol infusion. Following this EP study, RF catheter ablation (endo or endo/epi) was performed under sedation along with administration of high-dose isoproterenol. In a series of 16 ARVC/D patients, sustained VT was induced in 11 of the 16 patients (68%) during isoproterenol infusion, either spontaneously or by burst pacing. Furthermore, the morphology of the induced VT was similar to the baseline PVCs in 59% of the induced VTs. Based on the PVC/VT morphology, we performed a detailed map to identify regions of scarred myocardium demonstrating low voltage and multiple fragmented and delayed electrograms. The ablation strategy we employed was ablation of all of these areas. The endpoint of the procedure was noninducibility of VT and/or PVCs, and the isoproterenol challenge was repeated at the end of the ablation. Our results showed 85.2% cumulative VT-free survival after 1 year and 74.5% VT-free survival after 2 years. This reduction in VT recurrence also was associated with a decrease in PVC count among the ARVC/D patients.

Current Indications and Techniques for VT Ablation in Patients with ARVC/D

Catheter ablation now plays an important role in the management of our patients with definite or suspected ARVC/D. We generally recommend that a diagnostic EP study and endocardial VT ablation procedure be performed in patients who present with sustained VT with a left bundle block morphology and also in patients with a high frequency of PVCs (> 30,000 per 24 hours). For these patients, the EP study and endocardial mapping procedure is of value in confirming the diagnosis of suspected ARVC/D and also for risk stratification. If a single PVC or VT morphology is identified arising from the right ventricular outflow tract without evidence of endocardial scar, the diagnosis of idiopathic VT is supported. For these patients, a VT or PVC ablation procedure is often curative. On the other hand, if multiple morphologies of VT are found with evidence of endocardial scar, the diagnosis of ARVC/D is more

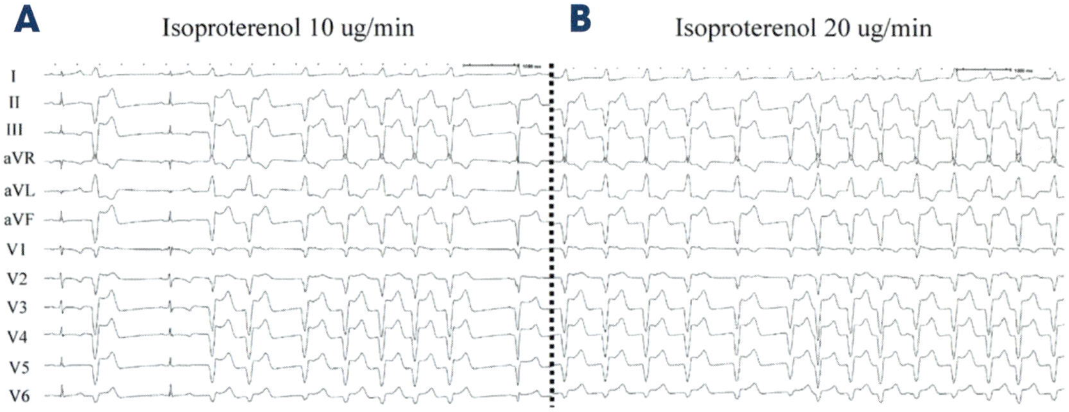

FIGURE 8.2 Complex ventricular ectopy during high-dose isoproterenol infusion (**Panel A**) that organizes into sustained monomorphic ventricular tachycardia (**Panel B**) in a patient with ARVC/D. *Source:* Philips B et al.[31]

likely. It is important to recognize that areas of low voltage may reflect scar but also may be due to poor tissue contact. The hallmark of ARVC/D is the identification of areas demonstrating low voltage as well as multiple sharp components of an electrogram (thereby also demonstrating slow conduction and areas of conduction block).

For most patients with a history of VT who are given a diagnosis of ARVC/D, we recommend placement of an ICD and drug therapy with a beta-blocker or with sotalol. If these medications are not tolerated or if recurrent VT develops, patients have the option of proceeding with a VT ablation procedure or being started on amiodarone. For those interested in VT ablation, a decision must be made as to whether their initial ablation procedure is endocardial only or if they prefer to undergo a combined endocardial/epicardial ablation procedure. Increasingly, we encourage patients with established ARVC/D who require a VT ablation procedure to undergo a combined endocardial/epicardial substrate-based ablation procedure. In more than 30 patients, our success rate has exceeded 85% with no serious complications.[30] Figure 8.3 shows a representative epicardial voltage map obtained from a patient with ARVC/D undergoing an epicardial ablation procedure. The endocardial voltage map in this patient was normal.

The epicardial ablation strategy, although associated with better outcomes, is not without potential for complications. Epicardial access technique requires considerable understanding of the cardiac and thoracic anatomy and, in our experience, preprocedural imaging to plan the access is crucial in avoiding complications. Structures that are at risk for injury are the liver, the stomach, the left internal mammary artery, the left lung, right ventricle, and the blood vessels in the interventricular groove. Laceration of vascular structures and perforation of the right ventricle often result in the need for urgent thoracotomy to achieve hemostasis.

We perform a contrast CT that is used to visualize pericardial fluid and for image integration to facilitate electroanatomic mapping. In the supine position, the pericardial fluid accumulates anteriorly and the heart sinks to the bottom of the pericardial sac. A shallow anterior approach targeting the mid-anterior RV wall is optimal for RV mapping and ablation. Axial and sagittal CT images will outline the pericardial

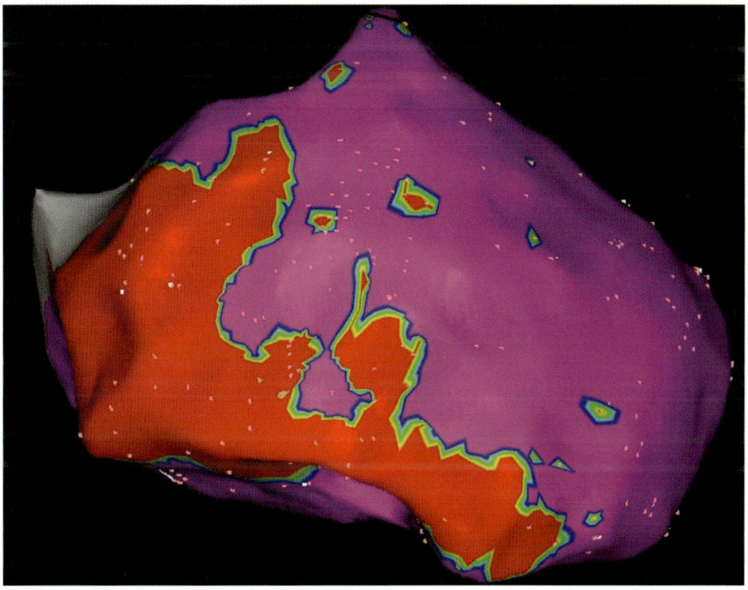

FIGURE 8.3 Epicardial 3D voltage mapping created on a Carto system demonstrating significant RV scar from the anterior to inferior RV extending from base to apex. Late potentials were also clearly present on the epicardial sites of scar.

space to be accessed, both providing the extent of the fluid and a visual guide to the depth and the distance from the midline. We perform our epicardial access under biplane fluoroscopy using anteroposterior and lateral views to emulate the axial and sagittal CT views. Using this technique, we have successfully performed epicardial access in 25 ARVC/D patients with no major complications except for mild pericarditis that resolved within 24 hours of the ablation.[30] After aspirating all the pericardial fluid, we routinely administer 125 mg of methylprednisone into the pericardial cavity before withdrawing the pericardial sheath.

We use a deflectable epicardial sheath in order to aid mapping of the RV and the LV epicardial surface. Using a 4 mm irrigated catheter, detailed mapping of the RV is performed while frequently aspirating the irrigating fluid in order to ensure proper contact of the mapping catheter. Interpretation of low voltage in the epicardium can be challenging, especially close to the atrioventricular groove and the apex, as the epicardial fat significantly attenuates the myocardial signal. Cut-off values for abnormal RV voltage that have been published, however, have not been extensively validated. For this reason, we rely on fractionated potentials that are distinctly later than the surface QRS, rather than low-voltage but early-activated regions. Fractionated late potentials are frequently observed in the perivalvular region, especially in the anterobasal and inferobasal RV. Both of these regions are affected in the majority of ARVC/D patients. We perform pacemapping to identify the exit sites of the induced VT, which often localizes to the region of late potentials. Systematic ablation of all the late potentials eliminates the PVCs and renders the VT noninducible.

Summary

In summary, catheter ablation of VT now plays an important role in the management of patients with ARVC/D. We recommend EP testing and a limited ablation procedure early in the course of the disease, especially in patients suspected of having possible idiopathic VT or PVCs. We also recommend EP testing and VT ablation using an endocardial/epicardial approach in patients with definite ARVC/D who have recurrent VT and have failed or been intolerant of antiarrhythmic drug therapy. A decision whether to undergo VT ablation is highly dependent on the experience of the operator and ablation center as well as the values and preferences of the patient who is contemplating the therapeutic options.

Conclusion

ICD therapy and catheter ablation are complementary strategies used for treatment of patients with ARVC/D. ICD implantation plays an important role for secondary prevention. It is also of value in ARVC/D patients felt to be at increased risk of sudden death based on careful risk stratification. Catheter ablation of VT in the setting of ARVC/D is an important palliative procedure, the goal of which is to decrease the frequency of VT episodes. As with all treatment strategies, a careful discussion with the patient is important in deciding on an optimal treatment strategy.

Acknowledgments

The authors wish to acknowledge financial support received by Dr. Calkins from the St. Jude Medical Foundation and Medtronic, Inc. The Johns Hopkins ARVC/D Program (ARVD.com) is supported by the Bogle Foundation, the Healing Hearts Foundation, the Campanella family, and Wilmerding Endowments, and the Dr. Francis P. Chiaramonte Private Foundation.

Abbreviations

EP electrophysiologic, electrophysiology
FFRW far-field R wave

ICD	implantable cardioverter-defibrillator
LV	left ventricle, left ventricular
MI	myocardial infarction
NSVT	nonsustained ventricular tachycardia
PVC	premature ventricular contraction
RF	radiofrequency
RV	right ventricle, right ventricular
VF	ventricular fibrillation
VT	ventricular tachycardia

References

1. Marcus F, Fontaine G, et al. Right ventricular dysplasia: a report of 24 adult cases. *Circulation.* 1982;65:384-398.
2. Corrado D, Basso C, Thiene G, et al. Spectrum of clinicopathologic manifestations of arrhythmogenic right ventricular cardiomyopathy/dysplasia: a multicenter study. *J Am Coll Cardiol.* 1997;30:1512-1520.
3. Dalal D, Nasir K, Bomma C, et al. Arrhythmogenic right ventricular dysplasia: a United States experience. *Circulation.* 2005;112(25): 3823-3832.
4. Marcus F, Zareba W, Calkins H, et al. Arrhythmogenic right ventricular cardiomyopathy/dysplasia clinical presentation and diagnostic evaluation: results from the North American Multidisciplinary Study. *Heart Rhythm.* 2009;6:984-989.
5. Sen-Chowdhry S, Syrris P, Prasad SK, et al. Left-dominant arrhythmogenic cardiomyopathy: an under-recognized clinical entity. *J Am Coll Cardiol.* 2008;52(25):2175-2187.
6. Dalal D, Tandri H, Judge DP, et al. Morphologic variants of familial arrhythmogenic right ventricular dysplasia/cardiomyopathy: a genetics-magnetic resonance imaging correlation study. *J Am Coll Cardiol.* 2009;53(15):1289-1299.
7. den Haan A, Tan B, Zikusoka M, et al. Comprehensive desmosome mutation analysis in North Americans with arrhythmogenic right ventricular dysplasia/cardiomyopathy. *Circ Cardiovasc Genet.* 2009;2:428-435.
8. Marcus FI, McKenna WJ, Sherrill D, et al. Diagnosis of arrhythmogenic right ventricular cardiomyopathy/dysplasia: proposed modification of the task force criteria. *Circulation.* 2010;121:1533-1541.
9. Buja G, Estes NAM III, Wichter T, Corrado D, Marcus F, Thiene G. Arrhythmogenic right ventricular cardiomyopathy/dysplasia: risk stratification and therapy. *Prog Cardiovasc Dis.* 2008;50(4):282-293.
10. Sen-Chowdhry S, Morgan RD, Chambers JC, McKenna WJ. Arrhythmogenic cardiomyopathy: etiology, diagnosis, and treatment. *Annu Rev Med.* 2010;61:233-253.
11. Boriani G, Artale P, Biffi M, et al. Outcome of cardioverter-defibrillator implant in patients with arrhythmogenic right ventricular cardiomyopathy. *Heart Vessels.* 2007;22:184-192.
12. Corrado D, Leoni L, Link MS, et al. Implantable cardioverter-defibrillator therapy for prevention of sudden death in patients with arrhythmogenic right ventricular cardiomyopathy/dysplasia. *Circulation.* 2003;108(25): 3084-3091.
13. Hodgkinson KA, Parfrey PS, Bassett AS, et al. The impact of implantable cardioverter-defibrillator therapy on survival in autosomal-dominant arrhythmogenic right ventricular cardiomyopathy (ARVD5). *J Am Coll Cardiol.* 2005;45(3):400-408.
14. Link MS, Wang PJ, Haugh CJ, et al. Arrhythmogenic right ventricular dysplasia: clinical results with implantable cardioverter defibrillators. *J Interv Card Electrophysiol.* 1997;1(1):41-48.
15. Tavernier R, Gevaert S, De Sutter J, et al. Long term results of cardioverter-defibrillator implantation in patients with right ventricular dysplasia and malignant ventricular tachyarrhythmias. *Heart.* 2001;85(1):53-56.
16. Wichter T, Paul M, Wollmann C, et al. Implantable cardioverter/defibrillator therapy in arrhythmogenic right ventricular cardiomyopathy: single-center experience of long-term follow-up and complications in 60 patients. *Circulation.* 2004;109(12):1503-1508.
17. Roguin A, Bomma CS, Nasir K, et al. Implantable cardioverter-defibrillators in patients with arrhythmogenic right ventricular dysplasia/cardiomyopathy. *J Am Coll Cardiol.* 2004;43(10):1843-1852.

18. Piccini JP, Dalal D, Roguin A, et al. Predictors of appropriate implantable defibrillator therapies in patients with arrhythmogenic right ventricular dysplasia. *Heart Rhythm.* 2005;2(11):1188-1194.
19. Bhonsale A, James CA, Tichnell C, et al. Incidence and predictors of implantable cardioverter-defibrillator therapy in patients with arrhythmogenic right ventricular dysplasia/cardiomyopathy undergoing implantable cardioverter-defibrillator implantation for primary prevention. *J Am Coll Cardiol.* 2011;58(14):1485-1496.
20. Bhonsale A, James CA, Tichnell C, et al. Risk stratification in arrhythmogenic right ventricular dysplasia/cardiomyopathy associated desmosomal mutation carriers. *Circ Arrhythm Electrophysiol.* 2013;6(3):569-578.
21. Epstein AE, DiMarco JP, Ellenbogen KA, et al. ACC/AHA/HRS 2008 Guidelines for Device-Based Therapy of Cardiac Rhythm Abnormalities: Executive Summary. A report of the American College of Cardiology/American Heart Association Task Force on Practice Guidelines (Writing Committee to revise the ACC/AHA/NASPE 2002 Guideline update for implantation of cardiac pacemakers and antiarrhythmia devices) developed in collaboration with the American Association for Thoracic Surgery and Society of Thoracic Surgeons. *J Am Coll Cardiol.* 2008;51(21):2085-2105.
22. Fontaine G, Frank R, Rougier I, et al. Electrode catheter ablation of resistant ventricular tachycardia in arrhythmogenic right ventricular dysplasia: experience of 15 patients with a mean follow-up of 45 months. *Heart Vessels.* 1990;5(3):172-187.
23. Fontaine G, Tonet J, Gallais Y, et al. Ventricular tachycardia catheter ablation in arrhythmogenic right ventricular dysplasia: a 16-year experience. *Curr Cardiol Rep.* 2000;2(6):498-506.
24. Ellison KE, Friedman PL, Ganz LI, Stevenson WG. Entrainment mapping and radiofrequency catheter ablation of ventricular tachycardia in right ventricular dysplasia. *J Am Coll Cardiol.* 1998;32(3):724-728.
25. Satomi K, Kurita T, Suyama K, et al. Catheter ablation of stable and unstable ventricular tachycardias in patients with arrhythmogenic right ventricular dysplasia. *J Cardiovasc Electrophysiol.* 2006;17(5):469-476.
26. Miljoen H, State S, de Chillou C, et al. Electroanatomic mapping characteristics of ventricular tachycardia in patients with arrhythmogenic right ventricular cardiomyopathy/dysplasia. *Europace.* 2005;7(6):516-524.
27. Verma A, Kilicaslan F, Schweikert RA, et al. Short- and long-term success of substrate-based mapping and ablation of ventricular tachycardia in arrhythmogenic right ventricular dysplasia. *Circulation.* 2005;111(24):3209-3216.
28. Marchlinski FE, Zado E, Dixit S, et al. Electroanatomic substrate and outcome of catheter ablative therapy for ventricular tachycardia in setting of right ventricular cardiomyopathy. *Circulation.* 2004;110(16):2293-2298.
29. Dalal D, Jain R, Tandri H, et al. Long-term efficacy of catheter ablation of ventricular tachycardia in patients with arrhythmogenic right ventricular dysplasia/cardiomyopathy. *J Am Coll Cardiol.* 2007;50(5):432-440.
30. Philips B, Madhavan S, James C, et al. Outcomes of catheter ablation of ventricular tachycardia in arrhythmogenic right ventricular dysplasia/cardiomyopathy. *Circ Arrhythm Electrophysiol.* 2012;5(3):499-505.
31. Philips B, Madhavan S, James C, et al. High prevalence of catecholamine-facilitated focal ventricular tachycardia in patients with arrhythmogenic right ventricular dysplasia/cardiomyopathy. *Circ Arrhythm Electrophysiol.* 2013;6(1):160-166.

9

Risk Stratification and Prognosis

Alessandro Zorzi, MD, and Domenico Corrado, MD, PhD

Introduction

Arrhythmogenic right ventricular cardiomyopathy/dysplasia (ARVC/D) is an inherited heart muscle disease, the clinical manifestations and natural history of which are essentially related to ventricular electrical instability. In particular, ventricular arrhythmias dominate the clinical scenario in the form of frequent premature ventricular beats, short runs of ventricular tachycardia (VT), or sustained monomorphic VT, predominantly with a left bundle branch block (LBBB) morphology. Such arrhythmias may provoke syncope, especially during physical exercise, and may degenerate into ventricular fibrillation (VF) leading to cardiac arrest and sudden cardiac death (SCD).[1-4] Only later in the disease, the progressive loss of myocardium may lead to severe dilatation and systolic dysfunction of one (usually the right) or both ventricles.[1,2] This chapter will address the mechanisms of SCD in ARVC/D, and the available tools to guide risk stratification and clinical management of ARVC/D patients.

Clinical Outcome and Sudden Death

The mortality rate of ARVC/D patients is currently estimated to be around 1% per year. Most deaths are related to life-threatening ventricular arrhythmias, which may occur at any time during the disease course. Progressive ventricular dysfunction leading to heart failure and embolic stroke may cause death in a smaller proportion of patients.[1,2] The overall incidence of SCD due to VF varies between 0.1% and 3% per year in adults with diagnosed and treated ARVC/D, although it is unknown and expected to be higher in adolescents and young adults, in whom the disease is clinically silent until sudden and unexpected arrhythmic cardiac arrest occurs.[5,6] Nava et al observed a lower mortality rate among family members during a mean follow-up of 8.5 years (0.08% per year) compared with ARVC/D probands.[7] Hulot et al[6] reported the long-term natural history of 130 patients with ARVC/D, who were referred to a tertiary center and followed for 8.1 ± 7.8 years. There were 21 deaths, which accounted for an annual mortality rate of 3% due to either progressive heart failure in approximately two-thirds of patients or SCD in one-third of patients.

The mechanism of SCD in ARVC/D is cardiac arrest due to VF, which frequently occurs as a first and definitive manifestation of the disease in young people without previous symptoms. In the early disease phase, VF may reflect acute ventricular electrical instability related to "hot phases" of the disease, with acute myocyte death and reactive inflammation, often characterized by dynamic T-wave inversion, ST segment elevation, and myocardial enzyme release. Older patients with a long-lasting disease more often experience scar-related, hemodynamically stable VT.[1,2]

It should be emphasized that ARVC/D shows a propensity for life-threatening ventricular arrhythmias during physical exercise, and participation in competitive athletics has been associated with an increased risk for SCD.[3,4,8] Identification of affected athletes by preparticipation screening has proven to result in a substantial reduction of mortality of young competitive athletes.[4] In addition, physical sports activity has been implicated as a factor promoting acceleration of disease progression. There is experimental evidence that in heterozygous plakoglobin-deficient mice, endurance training accelerated the development of right ventricular (RV) dysfunction and arrhythmias.[9] It has been advocated that impairment of myocyte cell-to-cell adhesion may lead to tissue and organ fragility that is sufficient to promote myocyte death, especially under conditions of mechanical stress, like that occurring during competitive sports activity.[2]

More recently, experimental animal models have suggested that gap junction remodeling and ion channel interference by the diseased desmosomes may be alternative substrates for anisotropic and delayed intraventricular conduction predisposing to lethal arrhythmias even in the prephenotypic phase of the disease, that is, before the appearance of histological fibrofatty substitution.[10-12] However, the clinical relevance of these findings remains to be proven.

Risk Stratification

SCD in ARVC/D patients is often an unpredictable event that occurs without alarming symptoms, and the only reliable strategy for SCD prevention is the implantation of an implantable cardioverter-defibrillator (ICD).[1,2] In recent years, a number of studies tried to identify the clinical variable associated with an unfavorable arrhythmic course. These studies suggested that symptomatic ARVC/D patients with prior cardiac arrest due to VF, a history of syncopal episodes, and sustained ventricular tachycardia (VT) benefit the most from ICD implantation. In contrast, the role of prophylactic ICD therapy in asymptomatic patients or relatives presenting with traditional risk factors such as a family history of SCD, severe RV dysfunction, and inducibility of sustained VT/VF at programmed ventricular stimulation (PVS) remains controversial.[13-41]

Previous Major Arrhythmic Events

In the series reported by Canu et al,[13] a prior history of aborted SCD from VF was documented in 2 of the 3 patients who died suddenly. In the DARVIN 1 study, Corrado et al reported that prior cardiac arrest due to VF and hemodynamically unstable VT are independent risk factors for life-saving ICD interventions in a large series of ARVC/D patients, while patients implanted because of VT without hemodynamic compromise had a statistically significantly better outcome, with a negligible incidence of VF episodes during follow-up (Figure 9.1).[14]

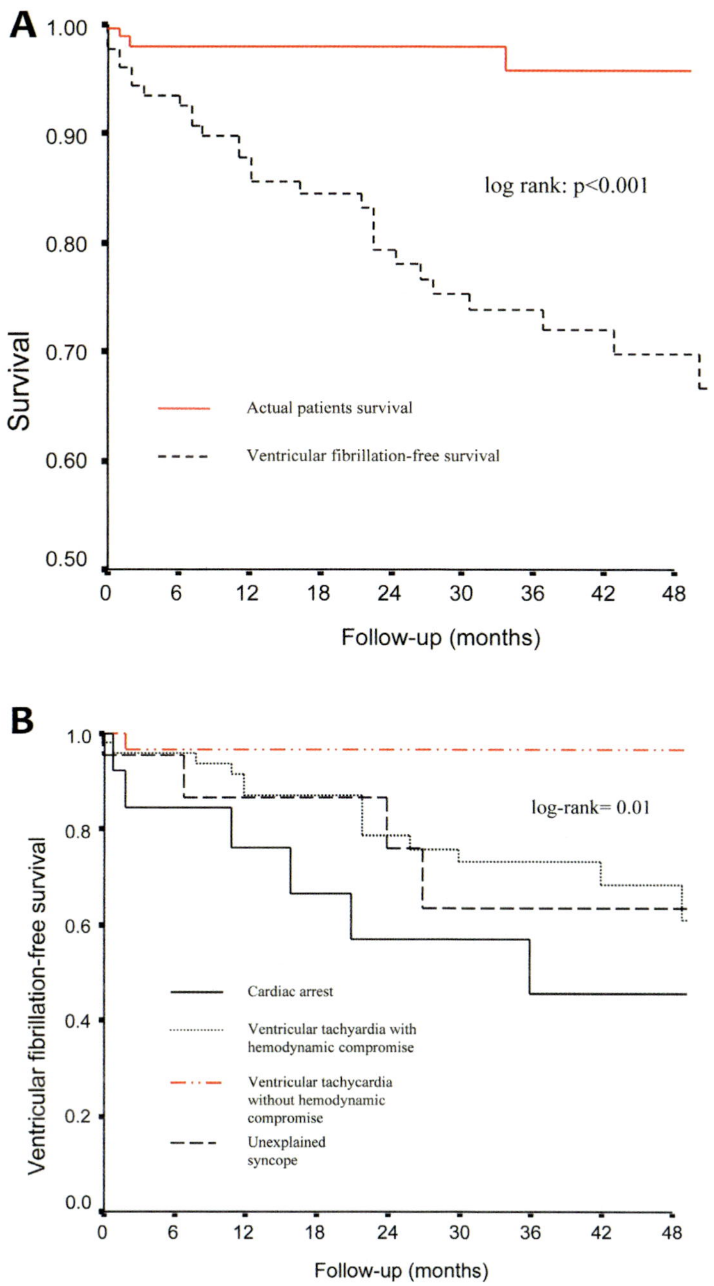

FIGURE 9.1 DARVIN I study, including ARVC/D patients who received an ICD for either primary or secondary prevention. **Panel A:** Kaplan-Meier analysis of actual patient survival (**upper line**) compared with survival free of ventricular fibrillation/flutter (VF/Vfl) (**lower line**) that would have been probably fatal in the absence of the ICD. The divergence between the lines reflects the estimated mortality reduction by ICD therapy of 24% at 3 years of follow-up. **Panel B:** Kaplan-Meier curves of freedom from ICD interventions on VF/Vfl for different patient subgroups stratified for clinical presentation. Patients who received an ICD because of sustained VT without hemodynamic compromise had a significantly lower incidence of VF/Vfl during the follow-up. *Source:* Modified from Corrado et al.[14]

Syncope

The importance of syncope as a risk factor for SCD in ARVC/D was first reported by Marcus et al,[15] and was later confirmed by other groups. Turrini et al[16] reported that syncope was an independent predictor of SCD with a sensitivity of 40% and a specificity of 90%. Among 15 ARVC/D patients reported by Blomström-Lundqvist et al,[17] a history of syncope was ascertained in all 3 SCD victims versus only 2 of 12 patients who survived. Nava et al[7] confirmed that syncope was the only clinical variable significantly associated with SCD in 19 ARVC/D probands, while it was never observed among 132 living relatives.

Syncope has been proven to be the strongest predictor of appropriate and life-saving device interventions in patients with ARVC/D who received an ICD for primary prevention (DARVIN 2). The 9% annual incidence of appropriate device discharges among patients with prior syncope is comparable to that observed in patients who underwent device implantation because of a history of cardiac arrest or sustained VT (Figure 9.2).[18]

Young individuals with genetic cardiomyopathies and/or ion channel disorders may suffer from vasovagal or, more widely, nonarrhythmic syncope, which makes differential diagnosis difficult and its prognostic value elusive. For instance, in patients with hypertrophic cardiomyopathy, several nonarrhythmic mechanisms such as reflex-mediated change in vascular tone or heart rate, left ventricular outflow tract obstruction, and supraventricular tachyarrhythmia may cause syncope. On the contrary, in ARVC/D patients, most episodes of syncope are secondary due to ventricular tachyarrhythmias and, thus, associated with a poor prognosis similar to previous sustained VT or VF.[18]

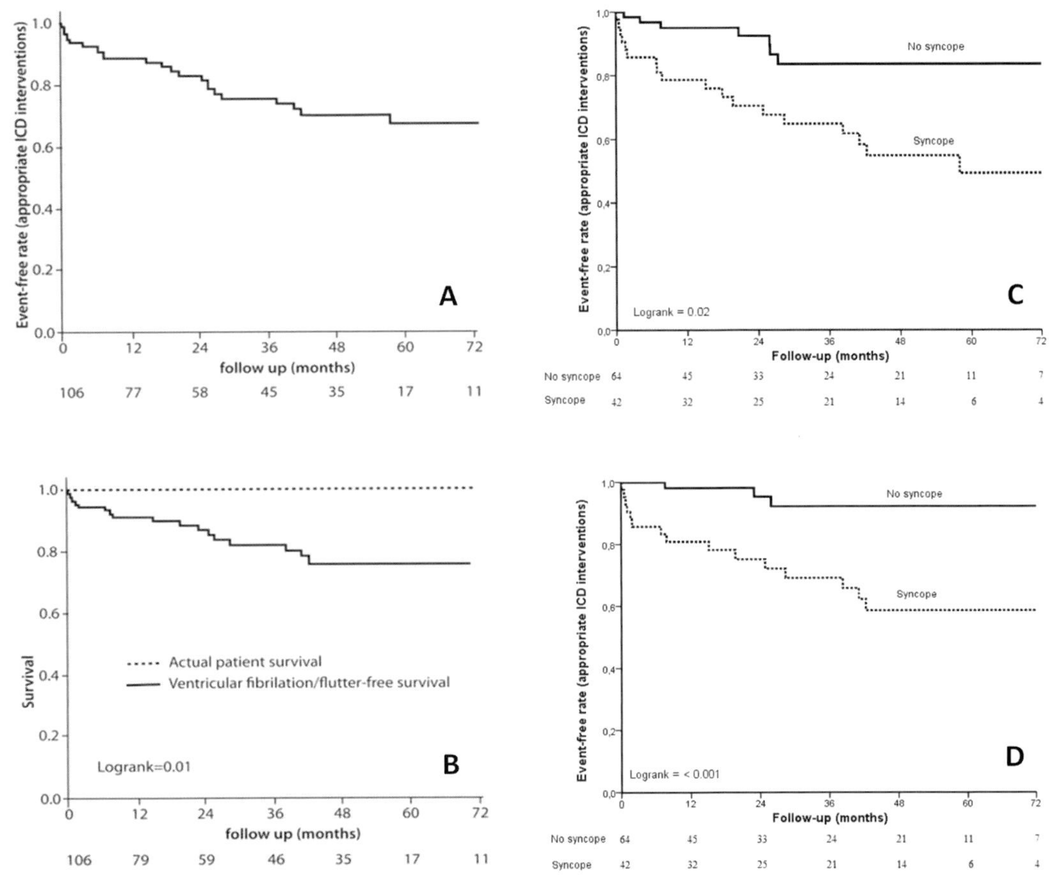

FIGURE 9.2 DARVIN II study, including ARVC/D patients who received an ICD for primary prevention only. **Panel A:** Kaplan-Meier analysis of cumulative survival from any appropriate ICD interventions. **Panel B:** Kaplan-Meier analysis of survival free of ventricular fibrillation/flutter (VF/Vfl) compared with actual patient survival. The estimated mortality reduction at 48 months of follow-up is 23% (ie, the difference between the actual patient survival rate of 100% and VF/Vfl-free survival rate of 77%). **Panels C** and **D:** Kaplan-Meier analysis of freedom from any appropriate ICD interventions (**Panel C**) and shock therapies on VF/Vfl (**Panel D**), stratified by syncope. *Source:* Modified from Corrado et al.[18]

Clinical Findings

ECG Depolarization Abnormalities. Right precordial QRS prolongation, QRS dispersion, and late potentials (LPs) on signal-averaged ECG (SAECG) are common depolarization abnormalities among ARVC/D patients and have been significantly associated with an increased arrhythmic risk. These ECG abnormalities reflect a right intraventricular conduction defect due to the fibrofatty replacement of the RV free wall, which may predispose to life-threatening ventricular arrhythmias.

Localized prolongation of the QRS complex in V_1–V_3 to more than 110 ms has been reported with a sensitivity of 55% and a specificity of 100% for the diagnosis of the disease.[19] QRS prolongation in the form of incomplete right bundle branch block (RBBB) or, more often, nonspecific conduction defects, is usually due to an intraventricular myocardial delay, also called parietal block. Incomplete or complete RBBB at the septal level may occasionally be the result of marked RV dilatation/dysfunction affecting the specialized right bundle branch (septal block). Right precordial QRS prolongation correlates with the arrhythmic risk as demonstrated by the study of Turrini et al,[20] in which patients who died suddenly showed a significantly greater QRS prolongation (125 ms) in V_1–V_2/V_3 compared with living ARVC/D patients with or without VT (QRS duration = 113 ms and 106 ms, respectively). In addition, they showed that QRS dispersion (the difference in duration between the longest and the shortest QRS intervals in the surface ECG) ≥ 40 ms, which reflects regional inhomogeneity of intraventricular conduction times and a delayed activation of the RV, was the strongest independent predictor of SCD in their cohort of 60 ARVC/D patients, with a sensitivity of 90% and a specificity of 77%. Accordingly, Nasir et al showed that a prolonged right precordial QRS complex with a delayed S-wave upstroke ≥ 55 ms is a significant predictor of severity and VT inducibility by programmed ventricular stimulation.[21]

In patients with ischemic heart disease, LPs on SAECG have been shown to be a noninvasive marker for areas of slow ventricular conduction, which is a prerequisite for reentrant arrhythmias. Several studies investigated the clinical meaning of LPs in ARVC/D. In the original series of Marcus et al,[22] among the 16 patients who underwent SAECG, 13 (81%) had LP. Blomström-Lundqvist et al[23] reported similar results with a 72% prevalence of LPs in their cohort of 18 ARVC/D patients. In the series of Wichter et al,[24] LPs were observed in 24 of 48 patients (50%), with a higher prevalence among those with a classic form of ARVC/D and more pronounced RV contraction abnormalities. Mehta et al[25] demonstrated a relationship between SAECG variables and the degree of RV enlargement. Although the SAECG appears to be a valuable test for diagnosing ARVC/D, the evidence of its utility for arrhythmic risk stratification is lacking. Blomström-Lundqvist et al[23] found that LPs were not predictive of ventricular arrhythmia in ARVC/D patients, as did Leclercq and Coumel,[26] who showed that the prevalence of LPs was similar in patients with or without sustained VT and their absence did not exclude the risk of SCD. Moreover, it was reported that repeated SAECG during follow-up did not appear to be useful in predicting the susceptibility to VT.[27] Turrini et al[28] demonstrated that, although LPs were univariate predictors of sustained VT, at multivariate analysis the only independent predictor of arrhythmic events remained a decreased RV ejection fraction. Furthermore, in patients with familial ARVC/D, an abnormal SAECG correlated with the severity of the disease, but not with ventricular electrical instability.[29] The predictive value of SAECG in this particular subgroup was low: only 44% of subjects with LPs had arrhythmias, whereas 76% with arrhythmias had abnormal SAECG. Likewise, the study of Nava et al[30] failed to show any correlation between SAECG and the risk of life-threatening ventricular arrhythmias.

ECG Repolarization Abnormalities. Several studies demonstrated that T waves in ARVC/D typically become negative as the disease worsens, and that a greater extent of negative T waves across the 12-lead ECG is associated with more severe RV dilation and dysfunction.[31-34] Turrini et al found that the incidence of negative T waves is higher among ARVC/D patients with a history of previous cardiac arrest or sustained ventricular tachycardia compared to those with a less severe arrhythmic burden.[20] Three recent studies extended this previous observation. First, Te Riele et al found that 88% of ARVC/D patients with documented, sustained ventricular arrhythmias within the last 6 months had an abnormal ECG. In particular, 122/145 (84%) subjects exhibited T-wave inversion in precordial leads (in 97 of them, extending to lead V_3 or beyond), while depolarization abnormalities such as Epsilon waves or terminal activation duration > 55 ms were present only in a minority of subjects.[35] Second, Bhonsale et al, focusing on desmosomal gene mutation carriers, found that the presence of T-wave inversion in ≥ 3 ECG leads was a powerful and independent noninvasive predictor of events during follow-up.[36] Third, Zorzi et al demonstrated that the extent of negative T waves was the only independent ECG predictor of the degree of fibrofatty substitution, as assessed by the endocardial voltage mapping (see below), and it prevailed over RV dilation and dysfunction in predicting the extent of the RV scar. In this study, the link between repolarization abnormalities and the underlying scar substrate was further substantiated by the association between the extent of negative T waves and the occurrence of major arrhythmic events during follow-up (Figure 9.3).[34]

Right Ventricular Dysfunction and Left Ventricular Involvement. A ventricular dilatation/dysfunction is a well-established clinical marker of a worse prognosis. In the study by Hulot et al[6] that tracked the long-term follow-up of 130 patients with ARVC/D, right heart failure and LV dysfunction were identified as independent risk factors predicting cardiovascular death. Peters et al[37] confirmed these results in 121 ARVC/D patients, in whom advanced RV dilatation/dysfunction and LV involvement were major clinical variables associated with an increase risk of SCD. Turrini et al[28] reported a significant association between a reduced RV ejection fraction (≤ 50%) determined by RV angiography and sustained ventricular arrhythmias. A number of ICD studies indicated extensive RV dysfunction as an independent risk factor for appropriate device discharges.[38,39]

Inducibility at Programmed Ventricular Stimulation

The electrophysiological study with programmed ventricular simulation (PVS) appears to be of limited value in identifying ARVC/D patients at risk of lethal ventricular arrhythmias due to a low predictive accuracy. The results of the DARVIN studies demonstrate that the incidence of appropriate and life-saving ICD discharges did not differ among patients who were and were not inducible at PVS, regardless of their indication for ICD implant.[14,18] Moreover, the type of ventricular tachyarrhythmia inducible at the time of electrophysiological study did not appear to predict the occurrence of VF during follow-up. These findings are in agreement with the limitation of PVS for arrhythmic risk stratification in other nonischemic heart diseases such as hypertrophic and dilated cardiomyopathy. In the study of Wichter et al,[38] VT/VF inducibility at preimplant electrophysiologic study

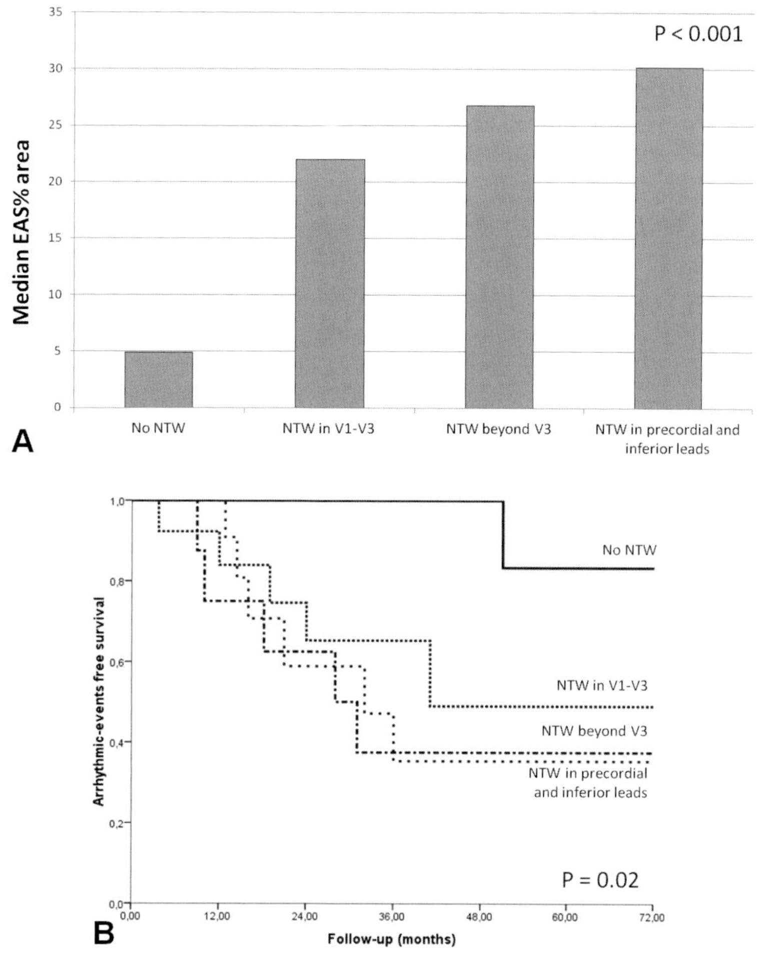

FIGURE 9.3 **Panel A:** Correlation between the extent of negative T waves (NTW) and amount of right ventricular electroanatomical scar size (EAS% area). **Panel B:** Kaplan-Meier analysis of survival free from major arrhythmic events according to presence and the extent of negative T waves. *Source:* From Zorzi et al.[34]

in ARVC/D patients with a previous history of cardiac arrest or sustained VT demonstrated just a trend toward statistical significance for subsequent appropriate device interventions. In addition, in 2 recent studies assessing the prognostic value of endocardial voltage mapping (see below), inducibility at PVS was a poor predictor of arrhythmic events during follow-up.[40,41]

At variance, inducibility at PVS was the most significant independent predictor of appropriate ICD firing in the ARVC/D cohort reported by the Johns Hopkins studies.[39,42] However, in the study by Bhonsale et al, the positive and negative predictive values of PVS inducibility were 65% and 75%, respectively, and a sizable proportion of patients experienced ICD interventions during follow-up despite a negative test. Discrepancies between study results may be explained by differences in arrhythmic endpoints (ie, life-saving interventions versus any appropriate ICD discharges), population characteristics, and stimulation protocols. In this regard, the predictive role of PVS inducibility as either a univariate or multivariate predictor of life-saving ICD discharges for VF/ventricular flutter was not demonstrated in the Johns Hopkins series.[42]

Electroanatomic Voltage Mapping

Electroanatomic voltage mapping (EVM) by the CARTO System allows identification and characterization (presence, site, and extension) of electroanatomic scars (EAS). EAS correspond to regions of ventricular myocardium that are characterized by a low electrical voltage, and may represent the substrate for life-threatening ventricular tachyarrhythmias. The technique has been demonstrated to enhance accuracy for diagnosing ARVC/D.[43,44] Recent studies prospectively evaluated the prognostic value of EVM in ARVC/D patients. Migliore et al[40] showed that an abnormal RV bipolar EVM and greater size of the RV electroanatomic scar predicted arrhythmia risk in their ARVC/D cohort (including patients with a previous episode of SCA, VF, sustained VT, and syncope), and appeared to be superior to traditional risk factors, including inducibility at PVS (Figure 9.4). In a highly selected small group of ARVC/D patients, all showing an abnormal bipolar EVM and receiving a primary prophylactic ICD, Santangeli et al[41] found that fragmented electrograms and delayed potentials recorded from the electroanatomic scar area were significantly associated with a greater incidence of appropriate shocks. It is noteworthy that in both Migliore's and Santangeli's studies, inducibility at PVS was a poor predictor of arrhythmic events during follow-up.

Molecular Genetics

At present, there is little evidence to support the use of genotyping for prediction of clinical outcome. Family screening for ARVC/D mutations may determine the genetic susceptibility of members, although it does not guarantee that disease will occur. Early identification of genetically affected individuals may raise complex management issues. A sizable proportion of gene carriers will not develop significant clinical manifestations because of the low disease penetrance. A large heterogeneity in clinical expression has been reported, which may be a result not only of different desmosomal gene defects, but also of different mutations within the same gene, compound mutations, and digenic disease. According to this marked variability of ARVC/D phenotype, the majority of relatives are likely to have a mild

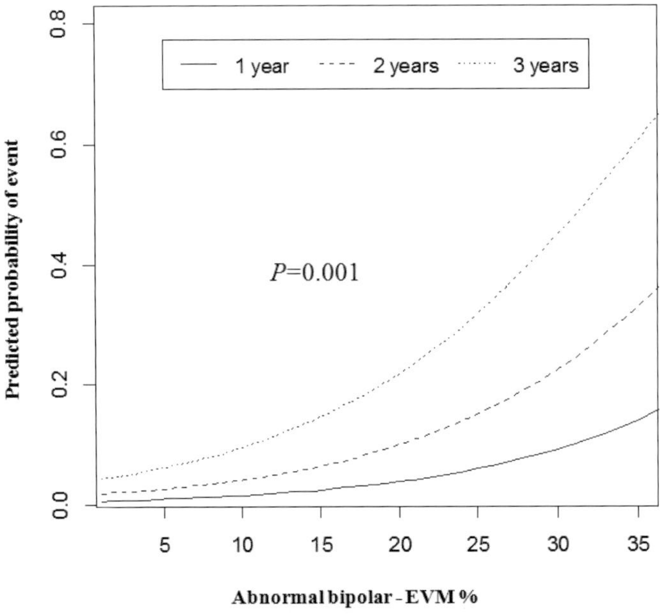

FIGURE 9.4 Predicted probability of experiencing major arrhythmic events at 1, 2, and 3 years on the basis of the extent of electroanatomic scar at bipolar endocardial voltage mapping of the right ventricle. The overall arrhythmic risk increases with percentage of abnormal bipolar-EVM (HR 1.7 per 5% abnormal EVM increase). *Source:* From Migliore et al.[40]

phenotypic expression and follow a benign course. On the other hand, patients may suffer arrhythmic events without warning symptoms and/or signs, in the setting of an unpredictable and abrupt acceleration of disease progression ("hot phases").[1,2]

Furthermore, genotype–phenotype correlation studies have failed to detect malignant ARVC/D mutations, which are specifically associated with an increased susceptibility to life-threatening arrhythmic events as to require prophylactic ICD therapy.[45] An exception is the study by Merner et al,[46] which reported a very malignant variant of ARVC/D linked to a transmembrane *TMEM43* gene mutation. No significant differences have been reported with regard to a series of clinical, ECG, and arrhythmic variables between ARVC/D mutation carriers and noncarriers. In addition, the proportion of patients who received an ICD and the incidence of appropriate discharges during follow-up did not differ between gene-positive and gene-negative probands, suggesting that genetic screening for ARVC/D gene mutations is unlikely to contribute significantly to arrhythmic risk assessment and stratification. These findings imply that other environmental or genetic factors, such as the presence of genetic modifiers or compound heterozygous mutations, may influence the severity of disease clinical expression.

Prevention of Sudden Death

Implantation of an ICD is the most logical therapeutic strategy for patients with ARVC/D, whose natural history is primarily characterized by the risk of arrhythmic cardiac arrest. Figure 9.5 shows the "pyramid" of arrhythmic risk stratification and indications for ICD implantation in ARVC/D patients, based on the annual rate of appropriate ICD interventions for life-threatening ventricular arrhythmias derived from observational studies.

There is general agreement that patients who survived an episode of VF or sustained VT most benefit from ICD implantation because of their high incidence of malignant arrhythmia recurrences.[14] On the other hand, asymptomatic patients had a favorable long-term outcome regardless of familial SCD and electrophysiologic study findings.[18] These results are par-

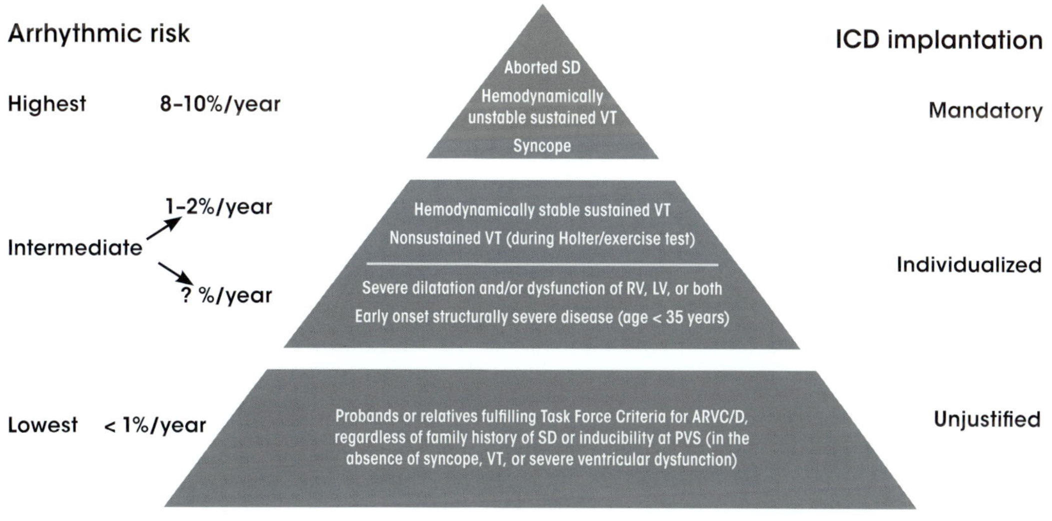

FIGURE 9.5 Pyramid of arrhythmic risk stratification and current indications for ICD implantation in ARVC/D patients, based on the annual rate of appropriate ICD interventions for life-threatening ventricular arrhythmias (ie, episodes of VF/Vfl) derived from observational studies. *Source:* Modified from Corrado et al.[47]

ticularly relevant for clinical management of the growing cohort of asymptomatic ARVC/D relatives and healthy gene-carriers, who are identified by cascade family screening. Finally, demonstration of nonsustained VT on 24-hour Holter monitoring and/or exercise testing in asymptomatic patients confers an increased risk of developing VT during follow-up, although it did not significantly predict the occurrence of potentially lethal VF/Vfl arrythmias.

In the absence of syncope or significant ventricular arrhythmias, it remains to be determined by further studies whether specific ECG abnormalities, severe dilatation and/or dysfunction of the RV, LV, or both, and early onset (age < 35 years) structural changes are related to an adverse arrhythmic outcome and require prophylactic ICD therapy. Moreover, the hypothesis that prophylactic beta-blocker therapy further lowers the rate of arrhythmic complications and slows disease progression remains to be proven. Finally, asymptomatic patients and healthy gene carriers should be prudently advised to refrain from practicing competitive physical exercise, not only for reducing the risk of ventricular arrhythmias, but also to prevent disease progression.[4,7,45]

Further investigations on larger ARVC/D patient populations with longer follow-up periods are warranted. This will refine the assessment of ARVC/D patients carrying a high SCD risk at preclinical/presymptomatic disease phases in order to optimize prevention strategies.

Abbreviations

ICD	implantable cardioverter-defibrillator
LBBB	left bundle branch block
LV	left ventricle, left ventricular
RBBB	right bundle branch block
RV	right ventricle, right ventricular
SCD	sudden cardiac death
VF	ventricular fibrillation
VT	ventricular tachycardia

References

1. Corrado D, Basso C, Thiene G. Arrhythmogenic right ventricular cardiomyopathy: an update. *Heart.* 2009;95:766-773.
2. Basso C, Corrado D, Marcus F, et al. Arrhythmogenic right ventricular cardiomyopathy. *Lancet.* 2009;373:1289-1300.
3. Thiene G, Nava A, Corrado D, et al. Right ventricular cardiomyopathy and sudden death in young people. *N Engl J Med.* 1988;318:129-133.
4. Corrado D, Basso C, Pavei A, et al. Trends in sudden cardiovascular death in young competitive athletes after implementation of a preparticipation screening program. *JAMA.* 2006;296:1593-1601.
5. Fontaine G, Fontaliran F, Hebert JL, et al. Arrhythmogenic right ventricular dysplasia. *Annu Rev Med.* 1999;50:17-35.
6. Hulot JS, Jouven X, Empana JP, et al. Natural history and risk stratification of arrhythmogenic right ventricular dysplasia/cardiomyopathy. *Circulation.* 2004;110:1879-1884.
7. Nava A, Bauce B, Basso C, et al. Clinical profile and long-term follow-up of 37 families with arrhythmogenic right ventricular cardiomyopathy. *J Am Coll Cardiol.* 2000;36: 2226-2233.
8. Corrado D, Basso C, Rizzoli G, et al. Does sports activity enhance the risk of sudden death in adolescents and young adults? *J Am Coll Cardiol.* 2003;42:1959-1963.
9. Kirchhof P, Fabritz L, Zwiener M, et al. Age- and training-dependent development of arrhythmogenic right ventricular cardiomyopathy in heterozygous plakoglobin-deficient mice. *Circulation.* 2006;114:1799-1806.
10. Sato PY, Musa H, Coombs W, et al. Loss of plakophilin-2 expression leads to decreased sodium current and slower conduction velocity in cultured cardiac myocytes. *Circ Res.* 2009;105:523-526.
11. Gomes J, Finlay M, Ahmed AK, et al. Electrophysiological abnormalities precede overt structural changes in arrhythmogenic right ventricular cardiomyopathy due to mutations in desmoplakin-A combined murine and human study. *Eur Heart J.* 2012;33: 1942-1953.

12. Rizzo S, Lodder EM, Verkerk AO, et al. Intercalated disc abnormalities, reduced Na(+) current density, and conduction slowing in desmoglein-2 mutant mice prior to cardiomyopathic changes. *Cardiovasc Res.* 2012;95:409-418.
13. Canu G, Atallah G, Claudel JP, et al. Pronostic et "evolution" a long term de la dysplasie arythmogène du ventricule droit. *Arch Mal Coeur Vaiss.* 1993;86:41-48.
14. Corrado D, Leoni L, Link MS, et al. Implantable cardioverter defibrillator therapy for prevention of sudden death in patients with arrhythmogenic right ventricular cardiomyopathy/dysplasia. *Circulation.* 2003;108:3084-3091.
15. Marcus FI, Fontaine GH, Frank R, et al. Long-term followup in patients with arrhythmogenic right ventricular disease. *Eur Heart J.* 1989;10(Suppl. D):68-73.
16. Turrini P, Corrado D, Basso C, et al. Dispersion of ventricular depolarization-repolarization: a noninvasive marker for risk stratification in arrhythmogenic right ventricular cardiomyopathy. *Circulation.* 2001;103:3075-3080.
17. Blomström-Lundqvist C, Sabel KG, Olsson SB. A long term follow-up of 15 patients with arrhythmogenic right ventricular dysplasia. *Br Heart J.* 1987;58:477-488.
18. Corrado D, Calkins H, Link M, et al. Prophylactic implantable defibrillator in patients with arrhythmogenic right ventricular cardiomyopathy/dysplasia and no prior ventricular fibrillation or sustained ventricular tachycardia. *Circulation.* 2010;122;1144-1152.
19. Fontaine G, Umemura J, Di Donna P, et al. La duree des complexes QRS dans la dysplasie ventriculaire droite arythmogene: un noveau marqueur diagnostique non invasif. *Ann Cardiol Angeiol.* 1993;42:399-405.
20. Turrini P, Corrado D, Basso C, et al. Dispersion of ventricular depolarization-repolarization: a noninvasive marker for risk stratification in arrhythmogenic right ventricular cardiomyopathy. *Circulation.* 2001;103:3075-3080.
21. Nasir K, Bomma C, Tandri H, et al. Electrocardiographic features of arrhythmogenic right ventricular dysplasia/cardiomyopathy according to disease severity. *Circulation.* 2004;110:1527-1534.
22. Marcus FI, Fontaine GH, Guiraudon G, et al. Right ventricular dysplasia: a report of 24 adult cases. *Circulation.* 1982;65:384-398.
23. Blomström-Lundqvist C, Hirsch I, Olsson SB, et al. Quantitative analysis of the signal averaged QRS in patients with arrhythmogenic right ventricular dysplasia. *Eur Heart J.* 1988;9:301-312.
24. Wichter T, Hindricks G, Lerch H, et al. Regional myocardial sympathetic dysinnervation in arrhythmogenic right ventricular cardiomyopathy: an analysis using 123I-metaodobenzylguanidine scintigraphy. *Circulation.* 1994;89:667-683.
25. Mehta D, Goldman M, David O, et al. Value of quantitative measurements of signal averaged electrocardiographic variables in arrhythmogenic right ventricular dysplasia: correlation with echocardiographic right ventricular cavity dimensions. *J Am Coll Cardiol.* 1996;28:713-719.
26. Leclercq JF, Coumel P. Late potentials in arrhythmogenic right ventricular dysplasia. Prevalence, diagnostic and prognostic values *Eur Heart J.* 1993;14:80-83.
27. Blomström-Lundqvist C, Olsson SB, Edvardsson N. Follow-up by repeated signal-averaged surface QRS in patients with the syndrome of arrhythmogenic right ventricular dysplasia. *Eur Heart J.* 1989;10(Suppl D):54-60.
28. Turrini P, Angelini A, Thiene G, et al. Late potentials and ventricular arrhythmias in arrhythmogenic right ventricular cardiomyopathy. *Am J Cardiol.* 1999;83:1214-1219.
29. Oselladore L, Nava A, Buja G, et al. Signal-averaged electrocardiography in familial form of arrhythmogenic right ventricular cardiomyopathy. *Am J Cardiol.* 1995;75(Suppl E):1038-1041.
30. Nava A, Folino AF, Bauce B, et al. Signal-averaged electrocardiogram in patients with arrhythmogenic right ventricular cardiomyopathy and ventricular arrhythmias. *Eur Heart J.* 2000;21:58-65.
31. Steriotis AK, Bauce B, Daliento L, et al. Electrocardiographic pattern in arrhythmogenic

right ventricular cardiomyopathy. *Am J Cardiol.* 2009;103:1302-1308.

32. Marcus FI, Zareba W. The electrocardiogram in right ventricular cardiomyopathy/dysplasia. How can the electrocardiogram assist in understanding the pathologic and functional changes of the heart in this disease? *J Electrocardiol.* 2009;42:136.e1-e5.
33. Nava A, Martini B, Thiene G, et al. Arrhythmogenic right ventricular dysplasia. Study of a selected population. *G Ital Cardiol.* 1988;18:2-9.
34. Zorzi A, Migliore F, ElMaghawry M, et al. Electrocardiographic predictors of electroanatomic scar size in arrhythmogenic right ventricular cardiomyopathy: implications for arrhythmic risk stratification. *Cardiovasc Electrophysiol.* 2013;24:1321-1327.
35. Te Riele AS, James CA, Bhonsale A, et al. Malignant arrhythmogenic right ventricular dysplasia/cardiomyopathy with a normal 12-lead electrocardiogram: a rare but under recognized clinical entity. *Heart Rhythm.* 2013;10:1484-1491.
36. Bhonsale A, James CA, Tichnell C, et al. Risk stratification in arrhythmogenic right ventricular dysplasia/cardiomyopathy-associated desmosomal mutation carriers. *Circ Arrhythm Electrophysiol.* 2013;6:569-578.
37. Peters S, Peters H, Thierfelder L. Risk stratification of sudden cardiac death and malignant ventricular arrhythmias in right ventricular dysplasia-cardiomyopathy. *Int J Cardiol.* 1999;71:243-250.
38. Wichter T, Paul M, Wollmann C, et al. Implantable cardioverter/defibrillator therapy in arrhythmogenic right ventricular cardiomyopathy: single-center experience of long-term follow-up and complications in 60 patients. *Circulation.* 2004;109:1503-1508.
39. Roguin A, Bomma CS, Nasir K, et al. Implantable cardioverter-defibrillators in patients with arrhythmogenic right ventricular dysplasia/cardiomyopathy. *J Am Coll Cardiol.* 2004;43:1843-1852.
40. Migliore F, Zorzi A, Silvano M, et al. Prognostic value of endocardial voltage mapping in patients with arrhythmogenic right ventricular cardiomyopathy/dysplasia. *Circ Arrhythm Electrophysiol.* 2013;6:167-176.
41. Santangeli P, Dello Russo A, Pieroni M, et al. Fragmented and delayed electrograms within fibrofatty scar predict arrhythmic events in arrhythmogenic right ventricular cardiomyopathy: results from a prospective risk stratification study. *Heart Rhythm.* 2012;9: 1200-1206.
42. Bhonsale A, James CA, Tichnell C, et al. Incidence and predictors of implantable cardioverter-defibrillator therapy in patients with arrhythmogenic right ventricular dysplasia/cardiomyopathy undergoing implantable cardioverter-defibrillator implantation for primary prevention. *J Am Coll Cardiol.* 2011; 58:1485-1496.
43. Corrado D, Basso C, Leoni L, et al. Threedimensional electroanatomical voltage mapping and histologic evaluation of myocardial substrate in right ventricular outflow tract tachycardia. *J Am Coll Cardiol.* 2008;51:731-739.
44. Corrado D, Basso C, Leoni L, et al. Three-dimensional electroanatomic voltage mapping increases accuracy of diagnosing arrhythmogenic right ventricular cardiomyopathy/dysplasia. *Circulation.* 2005;111:3042-3050.
45. Corrado D, Thiene G. Arrhythmogenic right ventricular cardiomyopathy/dysplasia: clinical impact of molecular genetic studies. *Circulation.* 2006;113:1634-1637.
46. Merner ND, Hodgkinson KA, Haywood AF, et al. Arrhythmogenic right ventricular cardiomyopathy type 5 is a fully penetrant, lethal arrhythmic disorder caused by a missense mutation in the TMEM43 gene. *Am J Hum Genet.* 2008;82:809-821.
47. Corrado D, Basso C, Pilichou K, Thiene G. Molecular biology and clinical management of arrhythmogenic right ventricular cardiomyopathy/dysplasia. *Heart.* 2011;97:530-539.

10

The Zurich ARVC Program

Ardan M. Saguner, MD

Introduction

Since the first systematic description of ARVC/D in 1977, numerous scientific contributions on ARVC/D have been made from individual research groups. Yet the need to establish national and international registries for ARVC/D to increase patient numbers at specialized centers in order to acquire knowledge and competence has been recognized in recent years, particularly after the publication of the Original Task Force criteria in 1994.[1-7] Importantly, our current knowledge concerning ARVC/D mostly originates from results of these well-established national and international registries (Figure 10.1, Table 10.1). In Europe, landmark scientific contributions came from France, Germany, Greece, Italy, the Netherlands, Scandinavia, and the United Kingdom. In 1992, Wichter et al from Germany published a large series on pharmacotherapy in ARVC/D, updated in 2005, and concluded that sotalol at a dosage of 320–480 mg/day was the most effective drug in suppressing ventricular arrhythmias.[8,9] In 2004, Hulot et al published a study on the clinical course of 130 patients with ARVC/D from a tertiary care center in France.[10] After a mean follow-up of 8 years, 14 patients had died due to progressive heart failure and 7 due to sudden death. The major cause of death was congestive heart failure and not arrhythmogenic sudden cardiac death, a finding highly attributable to appropriate ICD implantation in this cohort. Greek investigators found the association of ARVC/D with desmosomal protein abnormalities when they first described the link between cardiac and cutaneous manifestations in Naxos disease, so named because it was first reported on the Greek island of Naxos.[11] In Italy, an ECG-based preparticipation screening program for competitive athletes has been shown to be effective in detecting ARVC/D, with a reduction of mortality rates among young athletes in the Veneto region from 3.5/100,000 in 1979 to 0.5/100,000 in 2003.[12,13] In 2003, the DARVIN I study recruited 132 patients with ARVC/D from 22 institutions in northern Italy and 1 in the United States and found that almost 50% of the patients were saved by appropriate ICD therapy during the study period of 39 months.[14] In 2009, researchers from the U.K. found that cardiomyopathies are the most common cause of SCD in young British athletes, with ARVC/D attributed to 14% of these deaths.[15]

Besides Europe, other continents have also made important contributions to our understanding of ARVC/D. The South African ARVC (SA ARVC) registry was set up in 2004, and published its first results in 2009 on the clinical course of its cohort.[16,17] Although the characteristics of ARVC/D in South Africa are similar to the French cohort, the SA ARVC registry was able to identify 5 new *PKP2* gene mutations, with 1 gene mutation found in 4 different, unrelated Caucasian families. This has been explained as a founder gene effect, attributed to one of the early Dutch settlers arriving in South Africa. The genotypic profile of the SA ARVC cohort was in concordance with the genotypic profile of the Dutch cohort, published in 2006 and updated in 2011, in which *PKP2* gene mutations were found in more than half of all Dutch patients with ARVC/D.[18,19] Similar findings from separate cohorts from 2 different continents highlight the importance of historic, ethnic, and sociologic factors when investigating a genetically determined disease. A large ARVC/D registry from Johns Hopkins (Baltimore, MD) was established in the 1980s and has published numerous landmark papers since then.[20-26] In 2009, the Multidisciplinary Study of Right Ventricular Dysplasia Investigators, also from the United States, showed that amiodarone had superior efficacy in preventing ventricular arrhythmias compared to beta-blockers and sotalol in their North American cohort of 95 patients.[27] In

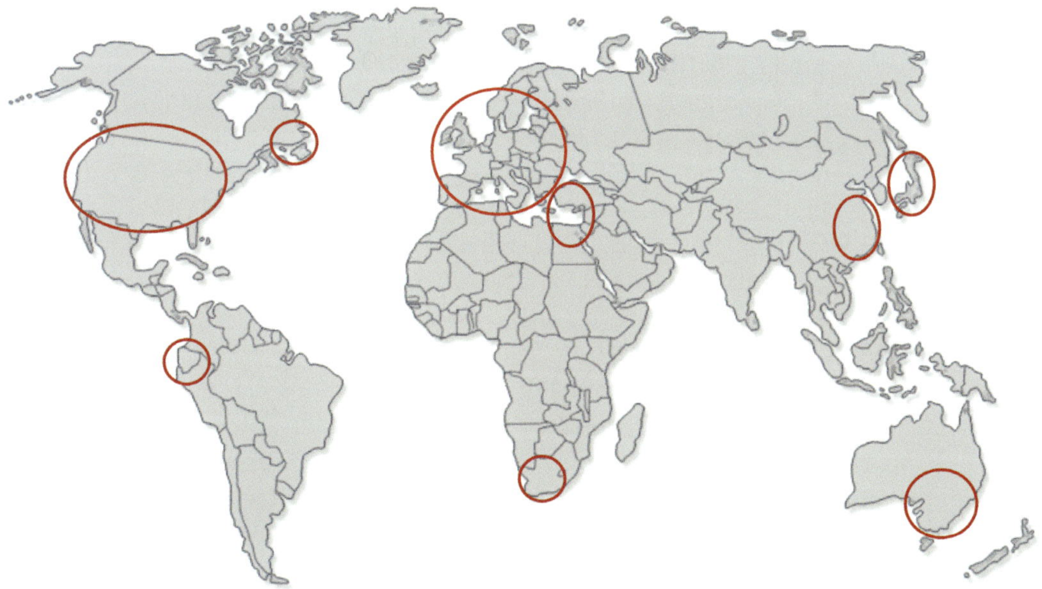

FIGURE 10.1 ARVC/D registries worldwide: For more than 15 years, ARVC/D has been studied in national and international networks in order to gather capacities and knowledge, and to increase patient numbers. *Source:* Adapted from Elmaghawry M, Alhashemi M, Zorzi A, Yacoub MH. *Global Cardiol Sci Pract.* 2012:26 (http://dx.doi.org/10.5339 gcsp.2012.26).

TABLE 10.1 ARVC/D registries worldwide

NAME	PATIENTS ENROLLED	FAMILIES ENROLLED	TYPE OF REGISTRY	STATUS	PROGRAM DIRECTOR	WEBSITE	CONTACT ADDRESS
The Johns Hopkins ARVC/D Program	1,226	226	Retrospective & Prospective	Active	H. Calkins, MD	arvd.com	ctichne1@jhmi.edu
Dutch ARVC Registry	491	93	Retrospective & prospective	Active	R. Hauer, MD	—	R.N.W.Hauer@umcutrecht.nl
Münster ARVC Registry	360	—	Retrospective & Prospective	Active	M. Paul, MD T. Wichter, MD		matthias.paul@ukmuenster.de
Nordic ARVC Registry	317	268	Retrospective & Prospective	Active	J.H. Svendsen, MD	arvc.dk	anders@kanten.dk
Zurich ARVC Registry	183	158	Retrospective & Prospective	Active	F. Duru, MD C. Brunckhorst, MD A. Saguner, MD	arvc.ch	arvc@usz.ch
Trieste ARVC Registry, Italy	129	—	Retrospective & Prospective	Active	B. Pinamonti, MD	—	dragosandreea82@yahoo.com
South African ARVC Registry	130	—	Prospective	Active	B. Mayosi, MD	www.paceafrica.org.za	arvc.sa@uct.ac.za
North American Multidisciplinary Study	101	—	Prospective	Inactive	F. Marcus, MD	arvd.org	fmarcus@shc.arizona.edu
Australian Heart Registry	87	40	Prospective	Active	C. Semsarian, MD J. Ingles, MD	heartregistry.org.au	j.ingles@centenary.org.au
Total	**3,024**						

Australia, a major national registry on cardiomyopathies was initiated in 2008.[28] ARVC/D has also been observed in Japan, China, and South America.[29-31] In 1998, investigators from Ecuador published a case series of 12 patients presenting with cardiocutaneous syndrome of palmoplantar keratosis and dilated cardiomyopathy resembling Naxos disease.[32] This syndrome is called Carvajal syndrome and has been attributed to severe desmoplakin mutations.[33] It is noteworthy that there have been case reports of patients with Carvajal syndrome from Turkey, Greece, and the Arabian Peninsula, demonstrating that cardiac genetic cardiomyopathies are not restricted to certain geographic areas.[34-37] As ARVC/D is present worldwide and does not have a specific racial or geographical predilection, international collaborations are of paramount importance to improve our understanding of this complex disease. To accommodate this issue, a multidisciplinary collaborative international registry has been established by the Study Group on ARVC/D of the Working Groups on Myocardial and Pericardial Disease and Arrhythmias of the European Society of Cardiology and the Scientific Council on Cardiomyopathies of the World Heart Federation in 2001, coordinated from Padua, Italy.[3] At the same time, the Multidisciplinary Study of Right Ventricular Dysplasia Investigators in North America was coordinated by Dr. Frank Marcus.[4] The comprehensive research of these large registries has laid the groundwork for the Revised 2010 Task Force Criteria for the diagnosis of ARVC/D.[38] Although our understanding of ARVC/D has significantly improved during recent years, numerous unresolved issues remain.

Establishment of a Swiss Registry

The Zurich ARVC Program was established in July 2011 and is based at the Cardiovascular Division of the University Heart Center, Zurich, Switzerland. The principal investigators are Firat Duru, MD, Corinna B. Brunckhorst, MD, and Ardan M. Saguner, MD, cardiologists with a special expertise in cardiac electrophysiology. The original idea for such a registry derives from the fact that the University Heart Center, Zurich—with initially more than 100 patients and family members—is caring for the largest number of ARVC/D patients in Switzerland, and thus shares a considerable expertise in this field. Yet, an important coincidence finally enabled the realization of this project. A young athlete and medical student from the University of Zurich experienced an episode of arrhythmogenic syncope while playing football at the age of 19. He was immediately referred to the university's hospital and diagnosed with ARVC/D, after he had been evaluated by several physicians in the previous years without a clear diagnosis being made. Subsequently, an ICD was implanted. As this young man's father was a leading member of the oldest and one of the largest Swiss private foundations, the Georg und Bertha Schwyzer-Winiker Foundation—an organization that supports social, cultural, environmental, veterinarian, and medical research projects, particularly at the University of Zurich—the foundation provided generous financial funding for the hospital's ARVC/D project, which gave birth to the Zurich ARVC Program. This program aims to characterize the Swiss ARVC/D cohort, based on various clinical and basic research protocols, in order to improve our understanding of this complex disease, but also to provide expert care for patients with ARVC/D in Switzerland. A nationwide registry is necessary to have an adequate sample size and prospectively evaluate the accuracy of clinical diagnosis, long-term clinical outcome, and efficacy of therapy. This registry has the potential to facilitate genetic and molecular research on the causes and pathophysiology of ARVC/D. Furthermore, availability of a national database will enhance awareness of this underrecognized but important disease among local cardiologists. Particular attention is drawn to genetic and molecular heterogeneity and joint genetic traits in comparison to other ARVC/D cohorts. To quote Guy Fontaine, the first describer of ARVC/D, "Switzerland is an interesting country with all its mountains and valleys, and it is worth investigating local genetic peculiarities of ARVC/D, possibly related to the fact that with this geographical and ethnical background, certain outstanding genetic variations may be found, similar to the Greek island of Naxos."

The Swiss people are usually physically active and many are engaged in sports activities; therefore, expression of the ARVC/D phenotype may result in more severe outcomes than in other cohorts around the globe. Ethical approval was obtained from the local ethical committee and prospective enrollment has been performed since July 2011. Physicians and other hospitals refer suspected cases to our local panel of ARVC/D experts, consisting of electrophysiologists, cardiac genetic specialists, cardiac imagers, heart failure specialists, and cardiac surgeons, for further evaluation. In addition, we have a very close collaboration with our cardiac pathology specialists and the forensic institute of the University of Zurich. Moreover, members of the local ARVC/D team regularly visit participating study sites to collect and manage patient data. All patients with suspected or confirmed ARVC/D are encouraged to participate in our registry. Written informed consent is obtained for DNA and RNA analyses from whole blood and tissue samples; release to the electronic registry, which is based on the internet platform secuTrial®; and storage of any biopsy material obtained during diagnostic workup. The functional organization of the registry has been formalized (Figure 10.2).[39] We have created our own homepage (www.arvc.ch), as well as our own logo (Figure 10.3), to increase the visibility of our registry.

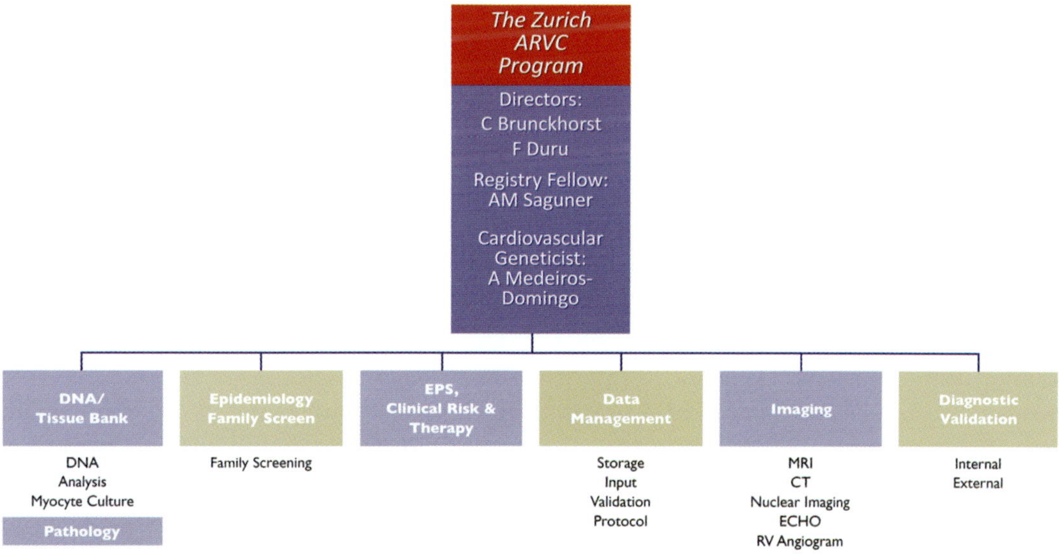

FIGURE 10.2 Organigram of the Zurich ARVC Program. *Source:* Adapted from *SA Heart.* 2008;5(4):148-154.

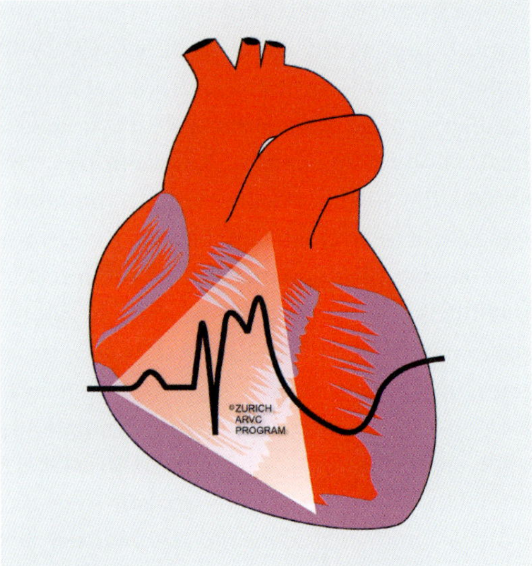

FIGURE 10.3 Logo of the Zurich ARVC Program.

Goals of the Swiss Registry

Our registry has 6 major missions:

- Genotype–phenotype correlations
- Identification of new genes and biomarkers
- Epidemiology
- Diagnostic validation
- Risk stratification
- Evaluation of therapy

DNA/Tissue Banking

Blood samples for DNA analysis are obtained from all index patients with a "borderline" or "definite" diagnosis of ARVC/D according to the 2010 Revised Task Force Criteria. At a later stage, we will also collect blood samples from "possible" cases with a family history of ARVC/D, dilated cardiomyopathy, or sudden cardiac death before age 35. After screening our samples for mutations in the 5 major desmosomal genes, *PKP-2*, *DSP*, *DSG-2*, *DSC-2*, and *JUP* (screening is currently being performed in the Institute of Human Genetics of the Universities of Zurich and Bern), we will extend our genome analysis to other potentially associated genetic loci. Next-generation sequencing will certainly enable us and other researchers worldwide to identify new genetic mutations and variations associated with ARVC/D in the future. Besides storage of blood samples in our –80°C biobank, we also store material obtained during endomyocardial biopsy or cardiac surgery.

Transcriptome analysis of myocardial tissue may help us to identify new genes and biomarkers involved in the pathogenesis of ARVC/D and overlapping cardiomyopathies. Transcriptome analyses are performed in collaboration with the Swiss Institute of Allergy and Asthma Research (SIAF) in Davos, Switzerland. Our extensive genetic studies with the target of at least 300 genotyped patients should enable us to draw meaningful conclusions about genotype–phenotype correlations, namely, to identify the influence of a certain genotype on the phenotype and clinical course of patients in the Swiss ARVC/D cohort. These correlations will contribute to improved diagnosis, risk stratification, and eventually targeted therapies. Besides genetic factors associated with ARVC/D, other mechanisms such as viral infection and autoimmune disorders are investigated in collaboration with the Laboratoire de Virologie Médicale et Moléculaire et Faculté de Médecine, Centre Hospitalier Universitaire, in Reims, France.

Epidemiology

The natural history of ARVC/D is still incompletely understood. Endogenous and environmental factors that lead to different forms of presentation such as sudden cardiac death, arrhythmias, and/or heart failure need to be investigated, particularly in different clinical ARVC/D subgroups and in as-yet asymptomatic family members. By means of ECG, signal-averaged ECG, exercise stress test, Holter ECG, echocardiography, cardiac MRI, right ventricular angiography, electroanatomical voltage mapping, endomyocardial biopsy, and genetic screening, we will establish a systematic epidemiological database of ARVC/D in Switzerland. Although a rare event, we are informed in case of an explanted heart due to ARVC/D obtained at cardiac transplantation, which constitutes a very valuable and informative source for experimental and clinical research.

Diagnostic Validation

With our registry, we aim to prospectively validate the 2010 Revised Task Force Criteria for clinical diagnosis of ARVC/D, specifically applied to our Swiss cohort. Detection of familial disease, particularly in young family members with less advanced disease, is a key task for all physicians who are involved in the care of patients with ARVC/D. Furthermore, development of improved quantitative methods to assess right ventricular but also left ventricular function and dimensions can help to enhance the specificity and sensitivity of ARVC/D diagnosis. Our recent and detailed echocardiography protocols include strain imaging, speckle tracking, and 3D echocardiography, and our modern MRI protocols include tissue deformation and evaluation of diastolic dysfunction for quantifying regional myocardial strain. Our recent voltage mapping protocol with the newly developed contact force catheter was applied to 15 patients so far. With these newer tools we hope to improve earlier disease detection, particularly in families without pathogenic mutations, and to add important data for a future version of the Task Force Criteria. Preliminary analyses of these data have shown that fractional area change (FAC) may be an important parameter of right ventricular function to predict adverse future events in ARVC/D.

Risk Stratification and Progress in Therapies

Important clinical markers of sudden cardiac death and a poor prognosis have been identified in recent years but are still incomplete—eg, the role of electrophysiologic study (EPS) for predicting future adverse events in ARVC/D is still controversial. We have recently published manuscripts demonstrating that inducibility of sustained monomorphic ventricular tachycardia, but also a history of heart failure and left ventricular involvement, may be helpful to identify patients who may need an ICD.[40-42] Although these were preliminary, rather small, and retrospective studies, we believe that EPS helps in risk stratification, and we hope to confirm these results in our prospective cohort with a larger sample size and less advanced disease. Based on future findings, we may identify antiarrhythmic drugs, heart failure therapies, and catheter-based therapeutic strategies to improve long-term outcome, while potentially reducing the number of ICD implantations in ARVC/D.

Conclusion

The Zurich ARVC Program represents the largest cohort of ARVC/D patients from Switzerland. It is our privilege that all 5 Swiss University Hospitals (Basel, Bern, Geneva, Lausanne, and Zurich) and many nonacademic Swiss centers already participate in our registry. Thus, we have been able to collect data from 183 patients with ARVC/D in the last 3 years. Despite the relatively short existence of our registry, considerable progress has been made with respect to patient recruitment and data collection. Our registry compares favorably with other ARVC/D registries.[16,25] The mean age of our cohort is 50.2 years with 128 male patients (70%), while 108 patients (59%) have an ICD implanted. Fifty-five percent of our patients have a "definite" diagnosis of ARVC/D according to the Revised 2010 Task Force Criteria (Figure 10.4), while the majority consists of index patients (n = 149, 81%). We have a large commitment for scientific collaborations. Cardiologists are requested to cooperate with us by referring index patients with confirmed or suspected ARVC/D for a second

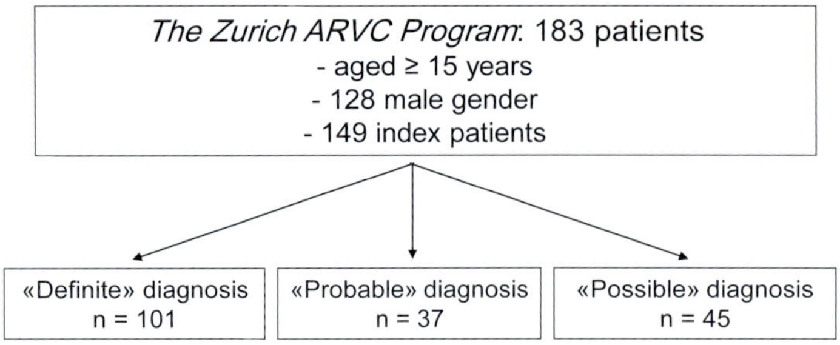

FIGURE 10.4 Classification of the Zurich ARVC Program patient cohort (October 2013).

opinion and/or enrollment in the registry and biobank. We consider cardiologic screening of all first- and second-degree family members of an index patient with ARVC/D to be of utmost importance to improve our understanding of this complex disease, leading to superior treatment strategies.

The need to establish national and international registries for ARVC/D to increase patient numbers at specialized centers in order to acquire knowledge and competence has been recently recognized. Our registry provides the potential to importantly contribute to this knowledge, to improve diagnostic accuracy, to better understand the natural history of the disease, and to optimize clinical management of our patients with ARVC/D.

Abbreviations

EPS electrophysiologic study
ICD implantable cardioverter-defibrillator
SCD sudden cardiac death

References

1. McKenna WJ, Thiene G, Nava A, et al. Diagnosis of arrhythmogenic right ventricular dysplasia/cardiomyopathy. Task Force of the Working Groups on Myocardial and Pericardial Disease and Arrhythmias of the European Society of Cardiology and of the Scientific Council on Cardiomyopathies of the World Heart Federation. *Br Heart J.* 1994; 71:215-218.
2. Corrado D, Basso C, Thiene G, et al. Spectrum of clinicopathologic manifestations of arrhythmogenic right ventricular cardiomyopathy/dysplasia: a multicenter study. *J Am Coll Cardiol.* 1997;30:1512-1520.
3. Corrado D, Fontaine G, Marcus FI, et al. Arrhythmogenic right ventricular dysplasia/cardiomyopathy: need for an international registry. Study group on arrhythmogenic right ventricular dysplasia/cardiomyopathy of the Working Groups on Myocardial and Pericardial Disease and Arrhythmias of the European Society of Cardiology and of the Scientific Council on Cardiomyopathies of the World Heart Federation. *Circulation.* 2000;101:E101-106.
4. Marcus F, Towbin JA, Zareba W, et al. Arrhythmogenic right ventricular dysplasia/cardiomyopathy (ARVD/C): a multidisciplinary study: design and protocol. *Circulation.* 2003;107:2975-2978.
5. Basso C, Wichter T, Danieli GA, et al. Arrhythmogenic right ventricular cardiomyopathy: clinical registry and database, evaluation of therapies, pathology registry, DNA banking. *Eur Heart J.* 2004;25:531-534.
6. Gjesdal K. Arrhythmogenic right ventricular cardiomyopathy—time for Nordic cooperation! *Scand Cardiovasc J.* 2008;42:363-365.
7. Fressart V, Duthoit G, Donal E, et al. Desmosomal gene analysis in arrhythmogenic right ventricular dysplasia/cardiomyopathy: spectrum of mutations and clinical impact in practice. *Europace.* 2010;12:861-868.
8. Wichter T, Borggrefe M, Haverkamp W, Chen X, Breithardt G. Efficacy of antiarrhythmic drugs in patients with arrhythmogenic right ventricular disease. Results in patients with inducible and noninducible ventricular tachycardia. *Circulation.* 1992;86:29-37.

9. Wichter T, Paul TM, Eckardt L, et al. Arrhythmogenic right ventricular cardiomyopathy. Antiarrhythmic drugs, catheter ablation, or ICD? *Herz*. 2005;30:91-101.
10. Hulot JS, Jouven X, Empana JP, Frank R, Fontaine G. Natural history and risk stratification of arrhythmogenic right ventricular dysplasia/cardiomyopathy. *Circulation*. 2004;110:1879-1884.
11. Protonotarios N, Tsatsopoulou A, Anastasakis A, et al. Genotype–phenotype assessment in autosomal recessive arrhythmogenic right ventricular cardiomyopathy (Naxos disease) caused by a deletion in plakoglobin. *J Am Coll Cardiol*. 2001;38:1477-1484.
12. Corrado D, Basso C, Pavei A, Michieli P, Schiavon M, Thiene G. Trends in sudden cardiovascular death in young competitive athletes after implementation of a preparticipation screening program. *JAMA*. 2006;296:1593-1601.
13. Corrado D, Basso C, Schiavon M, Pelliccia A, Thiene G. Pre-participation screening of young competitive athletes for prevention of sudden cardiac death. *J Am Coll Cardiol*. 2008;52:1981-1989.
14. Corrado D, Leoni L, Link MS, et al. Implantable cardioverter-defibrillator therapy for prevention of sudden death in patients with arrhythmogenic right ventricular cardiomyopathy/dysplasia. *Circulation*. 2003;108:3084-3091.
15. de Noronha SV, Sharma S, Papadakis M, Desai S, Whyte G, Sheppard MN. Aetiology of sudden cardiac death in athletes in the United Kingdom: a pathological study. *Heart*. 2009;95:1409-1414.
16. Watkins DA, Hendricks N, Shaboodien G, et al. Clinical features, survival experience, and profile of plakophylin-2 gene mutations in participants of the arrhythmogenic right ventricular cardiomyopathy registry of South Africa. *Heart Rhythm*. 2009;6:S10-17.
17. Hendricks N, Watkins DA, Mayosi BM. Lessons from the first report of the arrhythmogenic right ventricular cardiomyopathy registry of South Africa. *Cardiovasc J Africa*. 2010;21:129-130.
18. van Tintelen JP, Entius MM, Bhuiyan ZA, et al. Plakophilin-2 mutations are the major determinant of familial arrhythmogenic right ventricular dysplasia/cardiomyopathy. *Circulation*. 2006;113:1650-1658.
19. Cox MG, van der Zwaag PA, van der Werf C, et al. Arrhythmogenic right ventricular dysplasia/cardiomyopathy: pathogenic desmosome mutations in index-patients predict outcome of family screening: Dutch arrhythmogenic right ventricular dysplasia/cardiomyopathy genotype–phenotype follow-up study. *Circulation*. 2011;123:2690-2700.
20. Nasir K, Bomma C, Tandri H, et al. Electrocardiographic features of arrhythmogenic right ventricular dysplasia/cardiomyopathy according to disease severity: a need to broaden diagnostic criteria. *Circulation*. 2004;110:1527-1534.
21. Roguin A, Bomma CS, Nasir K, et al. Implantable cardioverter-defibrillators in patients with arrhythmogenic right ventricular dysplasia/cardiomyopathy. *J Am Coll Cardiol*. 2004;43:1843-1852.
22. Dalal D, Jain R, Tandri H, et al. Long-term efficacy of catheter ablation of ventricular tachycardia in patients with arrhythmogenic right ventricular dysplasia/cardiomyopathy. *J Am Coll Cardiol*. 2007;50:432-440.
23. Bhonsale A, James CA, Tichnell C, et al. Incidence and predictors of implantable cardioverter-defibrillator therapy in patients with arrhythmogenic right ventricular dysplasia/cardiomyopathy undergoing implantable cardioverter-defibrillator implantation for primary prevention. *J Am Coll Cardiol*. 2011;58:1485-1496.
24. Tedford RJ, James C, Judge DP, et al. Cardiac transplantation in arrhythmogenic right ventricular dysplasia/cardiomyopathy. *J Am Coll Cardiol*. 2012;59:289-290.
25. Bhonsale A, James CA, Tichnell C, et al. Risk stratification in arrhythmogenic right ventricular dysplasia/cardiomyopathy associated desmosomal mutation carriers. *Circ Arrhythm Electrophysiol*. 2013;6(3):569-578.
26. Kim C, Wong J, Wen J, et al. Studying arrhythmogenic right ventricular dysplasia with patient-specific IPSCS. *Nature*. 2013;494:105-110.
27. Marcus GM, Glidden DV, Polonsky B, et al. Efficacy of antiarrhythmic drugs in arrhythmogenic right ventricular cardiomyopathy: a

report from the North American ARVC registry. *J Am Coll Cardiol.* 2009;54:609-615.

28. Ingles J, McGaughran J, Vohra J, et al. Establishment of an Australian national genetic heart disease registry. *Heart Lung Circ.* 2008;17:463-467.
29. Ma KJ, Li N, Wang HT, et al. Clinical study of 39 Chinese patients with arrhythmogenic right ventricular dysplasia/cardiomyopathy. *Chinese Med J.* 2009;122:1133-1138.
30. Nakajima T, Kaneko Y, Irie T, et al. Compound and digenic heterozygosity in desmosome genes as a cause of arrhythmogenic right ventricular cardiomyopathy in Japanese patients. *Circ J.* 2012;76:737-743.
31. Ohno S, Nagaoka I, Fukuyama M, et al. Age-dependent clinical and genetic characteristics in Japanese patients with arrhythmogenic right ventricular cardiomyopathy/dysplasia. *Circ J.* 2013;77(6):1534-1542.
32. Carvajal-Huerta L. Epidermolytic palmoplantar keratoderma with woolly hair and dilated cardiomyopathy. *J Am Acad Dermatol.* 1998;39:418-421.
33. Norgett EE, Hatsell SJ, Carvajal-Huerta L, et al. Recessive mutation in desmoplakin disrupts desmoplakin-intermediate filament interactions and causes dilated cardiomyopathy, woolly hair and keratoderma. *Hum Mol Genet.* 2000;9:2761-2766.
34. Narin N, Akcakus M, Gunes T, et al. Arrhythmogenic right ventricular cardiomyopathy (Naxos disease): report of a Turkish boy. *Pacing Clin Electrophysiol.* 2003;26:2326-2329.
35. Bukhari I, Juma'a N. Naxos disease in Saudi Arabia. *J Eur Acad Dermatol Venereol.* 2004;18:614-616.
36. Antoniades L, Tsatsopoulou A, Anastasakis A, et al. Arrhythmogenic right ventricular cardiomyopathy caused by deletions in plakophilin-2 and plakoglobin (Naxos disease) in families from Greece and Cyprus: genotype–phenotype relations, diagnostic features and prognosis. *Eur Heart J.* 2006;27:2208-2216.
37. Ortac R, Tavli V, Diniz G, Yilmazer MM, Demirpence S. Naxos-Carvajal disease: a rare cause of cardiomyopathy with woolly hair and palmoplantar hyperkeratosis. *Anadolu Kardiyol Derg.* 2011;11:E17-18.
38. Marcus FI, McKenna WJ, Sherrill D, et al. Diagnosis of arrhythmogenic right ventricular cardiomyopathy/dysplasia: proposed modification of the Task Force Criteria. *Eur Heart J.* 2010;31:806-814.
39. Hendricks N, Mayosi BM, Okreglicki A. The South African Arrhythmogenic Right Ventricular Cardiomyopathy Registry: a brief report and a status report. *SA Heart.* 2008; 5(4):148-154.
40. Lemola K, Brunckhorst C, Helfenstein U, Oechslin E, Jenni R, Duru F. Predictors of adverse outcome in patients with arrhythmogenic right ventricular dysplasia/cardiomyopathy: long term experience of a tertiary care centre. *Heart.* 2005;91:1167-1172.
41. Schuler PK, Haegeli LM, Saguner AM, et al. Predictors of appropriate ICD therapy in patients with arrhythmogenic right ventricular cardiomyopathy: long term experience of a tertiary care center. *PLoS One.* 2012;7(9):e39584.
42. Saguner AM, Medeiros-Domingo A, Schwyzer MA, et al. Usefulness of inducible ventricular tachycardia to predict long-term adverse outcomes in arrhythmogenic right ventricular cardiomyopathy. *Am J Cardiol.* 2013;111(2):250-257.

Case 1

Difficult-to-Treat Arrhythmogenic Right Ventricular Cardiomyopathy/Dysplasia

Richard Kobza, MD, and Paul Erne, MD

Case Summary

The patient in this case was diagnosed in 1993 at the age of 38 with arrhythmogenic right ventricular cardiomyopathy/dysplasia (ARVC/D). During follow-up, he presented with recurrent ventricular tachycardia and heart failure due to biventricular involvement. He underwent medical treatment, repeated radiofrequency catheter ablations, and implantation of a biventricular implantable cardioverter-defibrillator (CRT-D); subsequently, he remained free of tachycardia from 2007 to 2013.

Case Report

In the winter of 1993, a 38-year-old post office clerk sought medical advice due to an episode of sweating and nausea during snow shoveling. The symptoms had persisted for 1 hour. After that episode, he felt well again and had no further complaints. The general practitioner observed a pathologic ECG (Figure C1.1) and referred the patient for cardiologic evaluation. Family history was significant; 2 cousins of the patient had died due to sudden cardiac death at ages 15 and 30, respectively. More than 50 members of his extended family were screened for the presence of ARVC/D; in the interim, another family member who had refused medical screening also died.[1]

In this patient, a 24-hour Holter ECG showed 4,300 premature ventricular complexes (PVCs), 440 couplets, 22 triplets, and 2 episodes of nonsustained ventricular tachycardia (VT). A transthoracic echocardiogram (TTE) revealed a normal left ventricle, but a dilated and globally hypokinetic right ventricle. The patient presented with an excellent exercise tolerance during stress testing, but several PVCs were noted during exercise. A coronary angiography showed normal coronary arteries. During electrophysiologic study, a sustained ventricular tachycardia with superior axis and left bundle brunch block morphology (240 bpm) was inducible. At this

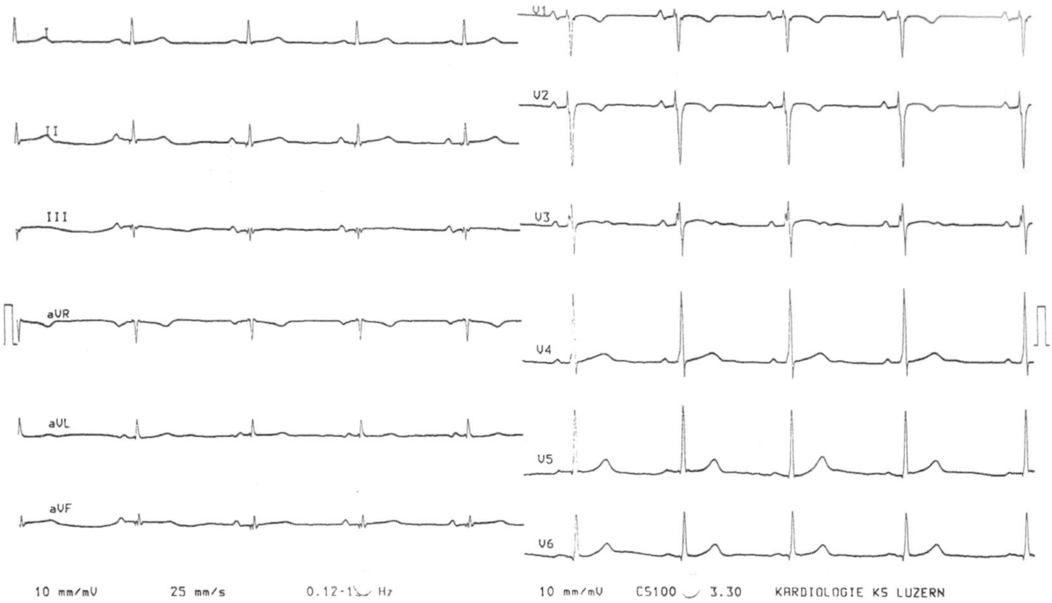

FIGURE C1.1 ECG showing terminal negative T waves in leads V_1 and V_2 and a slurred S upstroke in V_1.

point, the diagnosis of ARVC/D was made, and the initial symptom of sweating with nausea was interpreted as VT; thus, 1 major criterion and 4 minor criteria from different groups of the International Task Force Criteria for the clinical diagnosis of ARVC/D were fulfilled.[2] Treatment with sotalol (320 mg/day) was initiated. A follow-up 24-hour Holter monitoring under this medication showed no reduction of PVC load. During a repeat electrophysiologic study, a sustained VT with 240 bpm was again inducible under this treatment. The morphology of the induced VT corresponded to the VT found during the first electrophysiologic study.

Therefore, 1 month after occurrence of the first symptoms, the patient was referred a third time for electrophysiologic study; the PVCs were pacemapped and eliminated by radiofrequency ablation. Consecutively, sotalol was stopped. However, the patient reported 2 episodes of vertigo during follow-up that corresponded to sustained VT, and a second ablation procedure was performed 6 weeks after the first procedure. The VT targeted at that time showed a left bundle branch block morphology, with a slightly different axis than the previous VTs.

After the second ablation, no medical treatment was administered, and the patient remained asymptomatic for more than 1 year. However, in December 1994, recurrence of VT was documented, and sotalol (80 mg twice daily) was initiated. The patient experienced another 2 episodes of syncope that were both associated with insufficient medical protection due to irregular sotalol intake while traveling. In a follow-up TTE, an important progression of the disease was observed. The right ventricle was dilated, showing reduced systolic function, and additionally, mild left ventricular involvement was observed. Repeated Holter monitoring revealed 15 to 25 PVCs per minute.

As the ventricular arrhythmias could not be suppressed medically, the decision was made to initiate implantable cardioverter-defibrillator (ICD) therapy. The device, a Medtronic Jewel II 7219 (Medtronic, St. Paul, MN), was implanted under general anesthesia in June 1995. After ICD implantation, the patient reported an uneventful course and well-being under treatment with sotalol (40 mg twice daily) until October 1996. At that time, one appropriate ICD shock due to VT was noted. The VT occurred after the patient had stopped sotalol for 2 weeks without consulting his physician; therefore, medical treatment was reinitiated.

In 1999, ICD battery replacement was performed due to battery depletion (CPI/Guidant Ventak Mini 1793). In 2000, recurrent VTs were terminated by the ICD appropriately. An echocardiography at that time again showed a relevant progression of the cardiomyopathy. Both right ventricular and left ventricular systolic function were severely impaired. Medical treatment for heart failure was initiated, and the dosage of sotalol was increased to 320 mg per day. Under treatment with an ACE inhibitor, left ventricular ejection fraction increased from 35% to 48%.

In June 2001, an episode of strong malaise occurred such that the patient had to lie down and make an emergency call for an ambulance. The patient registered a VT with a heart rate of 150 bpm (Figure C1.2) that was below the VT detection zone of the ICD. As the patient became hemodynamically instable, an emergency cardioversion was performed. Interrogation of the ICD revealed 557 VTs that had occurred since the battery replacement in 1999. Of those 557 VTs, 75 had been treated successfully by the ICD. Consequently, the detection zone of the ICD was lowered and medical treatment was changed from sotalol to bisoprolol. Dosage of bisoprolol was increased stepwise up to 10 mg twice daily.

In September 2003, ICD replacement and upgrade to a DDD system was performed as the patient presented with progressive heart failure, chronotropic incompetence under beta-blockade, and ICD battery depletion. The course from September 2003 to June 2005 was uneventful; the patient presented with stable dyspnea NYHA II without any tachycardia.

In July 2005, recurrence of symptomatic VTs at a heart rate of 136 bpm (Figure C1.3) was observed. During tachycardia, the patient felt dizzy und unwell. The tachycardias were self-limiting, and occurrence was triggered by alcohol intake. However, in March 2006, this slow VT did not terminate spontaneously, and the patient had to be hospitalized. The tachycardia remained incessant, despite initiation of treatment with amiodarone. Therefore, the patient was referred for repeat radiofrequency ablation. In the electrophysiology lab, a VT at a heart rate of 120 bpm was documented (Figure C1.4). After activation and voltage mapping (Figure C1.5), radiofrequency ablation was performed with an irrigated tip catheter. After successful ablation treatment with a beta-blocker, amiodarone and an ACE inhibitor was continued. An echocardiogram performed in May 2007 showed severely impaired right and left ventricular systolic function and significant inter- and intraventricular dyssynchrony. Therefore, the decision to perform an upgrade to a biventricular ICD (CRT-D) was made in October 2007. The implantation of the left

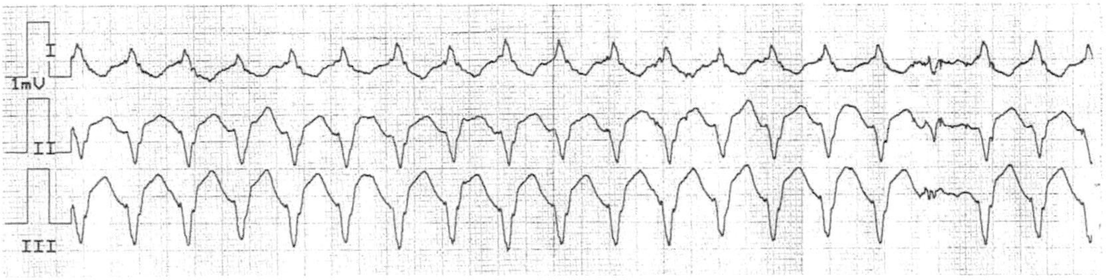

FIGURE C1.2 ECG strip showing ventricular tachycardia at a heart rate of 150 bpm with one fusion beat.

ventricular lead (Figure C1.6) was performed epicardially by lateral thoracotomy (endocardial implantation was not possible at that time due to technical problems in the cathlab). Under biventricular pacing, the patient was stable and presented with dyspnea NYHA II. The echocardiographic findings remained stable (Figure C1.7). During follow-up from 2007 to 2013, no VTs were registered by the device, and the patient was able to perform his job as a post office clerk. Over the years, the electrical measurements of the device showed a decline of sensing function and a rise in ventricular threshold (Table C1.1), both of which may have been a consequence of progressive fibrofatty infiltration of the right ventricle.

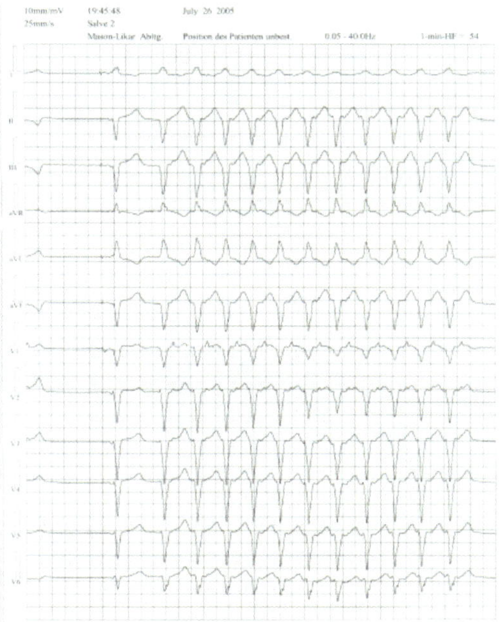

FIGURE C1.3 A 12-lead ECG showing a ventricular tachycardia at a heart rate of 136 bpm with left bundle branch block morphology, a superior axis, and negative concordance in V_1 to V_6.

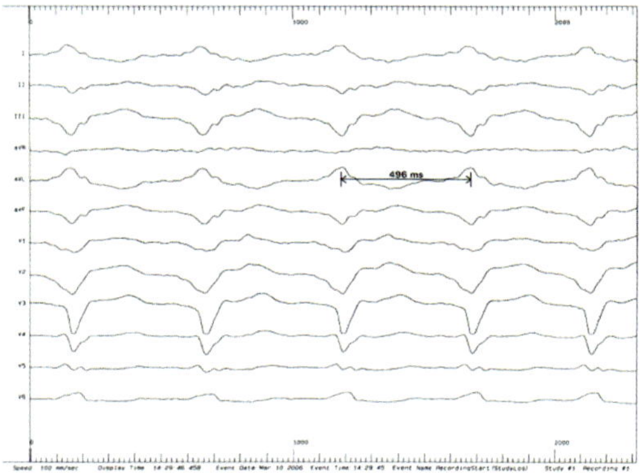

FIGURE C1.4 Ventricular tachycardia at a heart rate of 120 bpm registered in the electrophysiology lab. The VT has left bundle branch block morphology, a superior axis, and R/S transition in V_4/V_5.

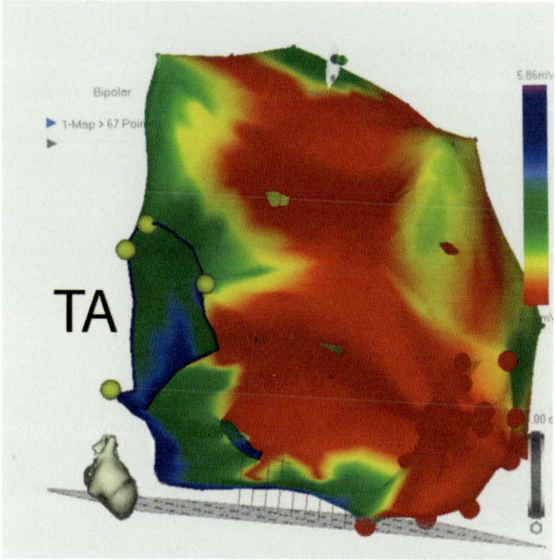

FIGURE C1.5 3D endocardial voltage map of the right ventricle in a modified right lateral view. Red zones correspond to low-voltage areas; red dots show ablation points. TA = tricuspid annulus.

TABLE C1.1 Change of sensitivity and ventricular threshold

	1995	1996	2000	2003	2006	2008	2010	2012
R-WAVE (mV)	5.5	5.5	6.6	4.7	4.4	3.5	3.3	3.3
THRESHOLD V/ms	2.8/0.1	2.8/0.1	1.1/0.5	1.0/0.5	0.7/0.5	1.2/0.5	1.5/0.5	1.6/0.5

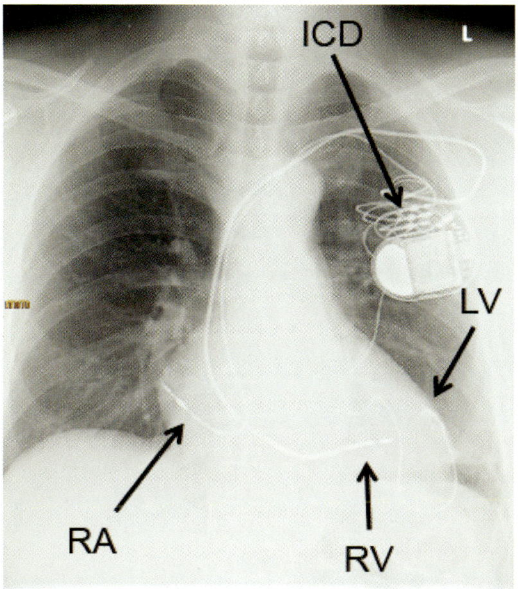

FIGURE C1.6 Postero-anterior chest radiography. Implantable cardioverter-defibrillator (ICD) is implanted in the upper left infraclavicular region. The atrial lead (RA) is visible in the right lateral atrial wall, and one ventricular lead (RV) is visible in the right ventricular apex. The left ventricular lead (LV) is implanted epicardially.

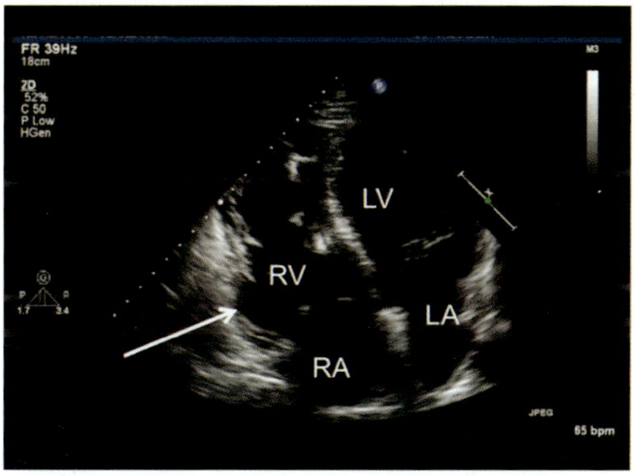

FIGURE C1.7 Transthoracic echocardiogram (apical 4-chamber view). The right ventricle (RV) and right atrium are enlarged and the RV presents with a paper-thin free wall; arrow depicts subtricuspid aneurysm. LV = left ventricle; RA = right atrium; RV = right ventricle.

Conclusion

This case illustrates the nature of ARVC/D as a progressive disease with hereditary transmission. Often, aggressive treatment is needed, including long-acting beta-blockers, sotalol or amiodarone, and heart failure medication. With optimal medical treatment, devices, and radiofrequency ablation, a favorable course with a good quality of life may be achieved, even in severe, progressive forms with biventricular involvement, as presented in this case.

Abbreviations

ICD implantable cardioverter-defibrillator
PVC premature ventricular contraction
VT ventricular tachycardia

References

1. Rampazzo A, Nava A, Erne P et al. A new locus for arrhythmogenic right ventricular cardiomyopathy (ARVD2) maps to chromosome 1q42-q43. *Hum Molec Genet.* 1995;4:2151-2154.
2. Marcus FI, McKenna WJ, Sherrill D, et al. Diagnosis of arrhythmogenic right ventricular cardiomyopathy/dysplasia: proposed modification of the Task Force Criteria. *Eur Heart J.* 2010 Apr;31(7):806-814.

Case 2

Arrhythmogenic Right Ventricular Cardiomyopathy/Dysplasia in Sports: Rare Incident or the "Tip of the Iceberg"?

Christian M. Schmied, MD

Case Summary

The patient in this case, a 16-year-old female, presented with complaint of near-syncope associated with sports activity. Emergent examination found her to be hypotensive with an elevated heart rate. Findings from 12-lead ECG and transthoracic echocardiogram offered a definitive diagnosis of ARVC/D. The patient subsequently received a dual-chamber implantable cardioverter-defibrillator (ICD) device and was restricted from participation in competitive sports.

Case Report

A previously healthy 16-year-old female floorball player experienced an episode of sudden-onset general weakness and lightheadedness in the middle of a Sunday afternoon game. She went to the sideline and complained of "near fainting," so her coach immediately called an ambulance, which brought her to our emergency department. We found a conscious but compromised young athlete in a reduced mental state. Blood pressure measurements on both arms showed hypotensive values of 100/60 mmHg; palpatory central and peripheral pulse wave appeared blunted, and heart rate was higher than 160 bpm.

A 12-lead resting electrocardiogram (ECG) was performed (Figure C2.1). The ECG demonstrated a regular, wide-complex tachycardia with left bundle branch block morphology, superior axis, and atrioventricular dissociation consistent with ventricular tachycardia (VT) originating from the inferior right ventricle (RV). Due to hemodynamic instability, synchronized electrocardioversion was performed immediately, resulting in prompt cessation of the tachycardia, associated with rapid improvement of vital signs and general physical status.

On the subsequent ECG, regular sinus rhythm was noted, with slightly widened QRS complexes, a slurred S upstroke, and deep T-wave inversion in the right precordial leads

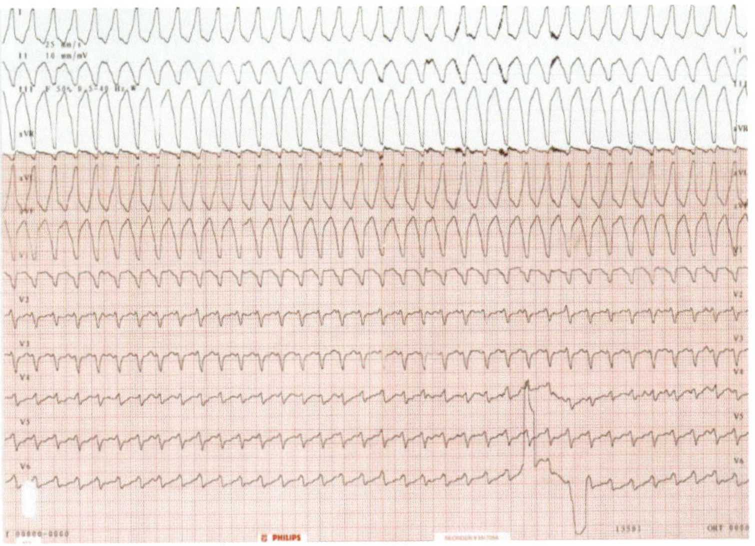

FIGURE C2.1 The patient's 12-lead resting ECG at admission showing wide-complex tachycardia with a left bundle branch morphology and superior axis.

(V_1 to V_3) (Figure C2.2). The findings offered a strong suspicion of first manifestation of arrhythmogenic right ventricular cardiomyopathy/dysplasia (ARVC/D), so a transthoracic echocardiography was performed (Figure C2.3). The echocardiogram showed RV dilatation and aneurysmatic changes in segments of the RV wall. Thus, the diagnosis of definite ARVC/D was confirmed by the presence of 4 criteria: 1 major arrhythmia criterion, 1 major repolarization criterion, 1 major imaging criterion, and 1 minor depolarization criterion.

The young athlete rapidly recovered and subsequently underwent implantation of a dual-chamber ICD. Thereafter, she was restricted from competitive sports, with the possible exception of low dynamic/low static sports (such as billiards, bowling, or golf).[1,2]

Discussion

This case report exemplifies some of the crucial issues in the spectrum of ARVC/D in sports. When Corrado and colleagues published their landmark and groundbreaking assessment of 269 young competitive athletes

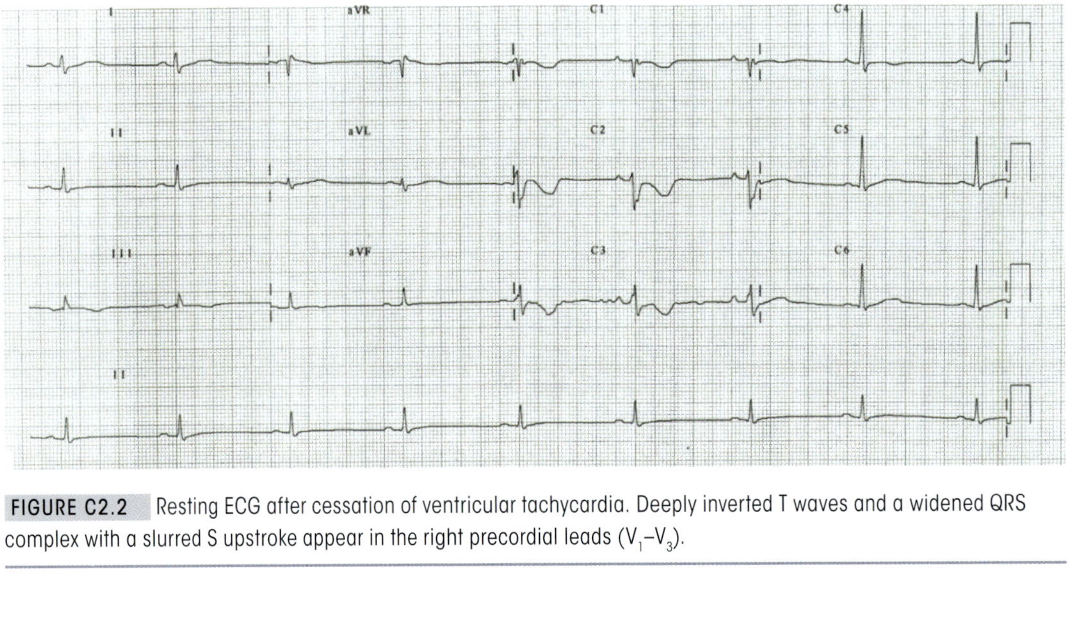

FIGURE C2.2 Resting ECG after cessation of ventricular tachycardia. Deeply inverted T waves and a widened QRS complex with a slurred S upstroke appear in the right precordial leads (V_1–V_3).

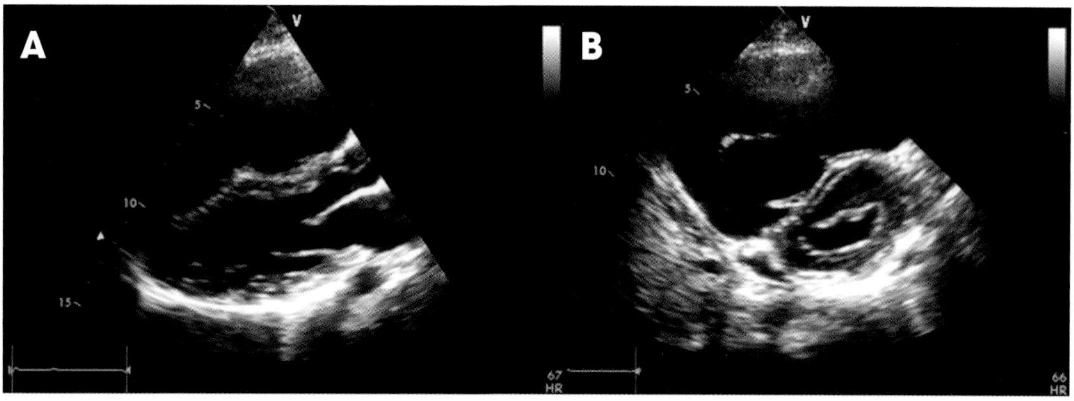

FIGURE C2.3 Parasternal long (**A**) and short axis (**B**) views showing massive right ventricular (RV) dilatation.

who suddenly died during sports,[3,4] ARVC/D immediately gained closer scrutiny among sports cardiologists because 22.4% of sudden cardiac deaths (SCD) in this cohort of young athletes were due to ARVC/D, making it the most common cause.[3,4] This was surprising, as the disease was not of relevant prevalence in former surveys that examined these tragic sports-related events in competitive North American athletes.[5-7] Yet the reasons for this unexpectedly high rate of SCD due to ARVC/D in the Italian survey are a matter of ongoing debate: It is a well-recognized fact that in a normal population, ARVC/D has been underdiagnosed in recent reports and, consequently, must be a relevant issue in competitive athletes as well.[3,4,8,9]

Frequently, the first overt clinical manifestation of the disease in athletes is sudden cardiac arrest (SCA) during intensive activity, as preceding and suggestive symptoms are mostly unspecific.[3,10] Corrado et al demonstrated that syncope and palpitations on exertion appeared in about half of the affected athletes with underlying ARVC/D prior to a fatal cardiac event.[3] For example, the young female floorball player in this case retrospectively mentioned only nonspecific symptoms as transient fatigue and mild dizziness at times.

Nevertheless, use of the 12-lead ECG has considerably improved the accuracy of detection of this fatal disease in athletes.[8,11-18] With a high diagnostic sensitivity and specificity (up to 71% and 96%, respectively), it has become the major diagnostic tool in primary screening of young athletes.[19,20]

There are only few differential diagnoses of this ECG pattern in athletes. Particularly, the so called "Afro-Caribbean" early repolarization pattern—a mostly benign finding with T-wave inversions in the anterior leads that are characteristically associated with a preceding convex "domed" ST-segment elevation—has recently gained growing attention (Figure C2.4).[13,16,21-23]

Since SCA and SCD became a major public issue—not only in young competitive athletes but in the general population as well—ambitious strategies were established to prevent these fatal events in athletes.[11,12,24] Currently, the feasibility and accuracy of 2 main strategies are the matter of debate: First, primarily in North America, expert panels recommend a baseline screening integrating a focused physical examination in combination with a questionnaire assessing the athletes' personal and family history.[12] Second, the European approach, based on mainly Italian data and incorporated by the European Society of Cardiology (ESC), the International Olympic

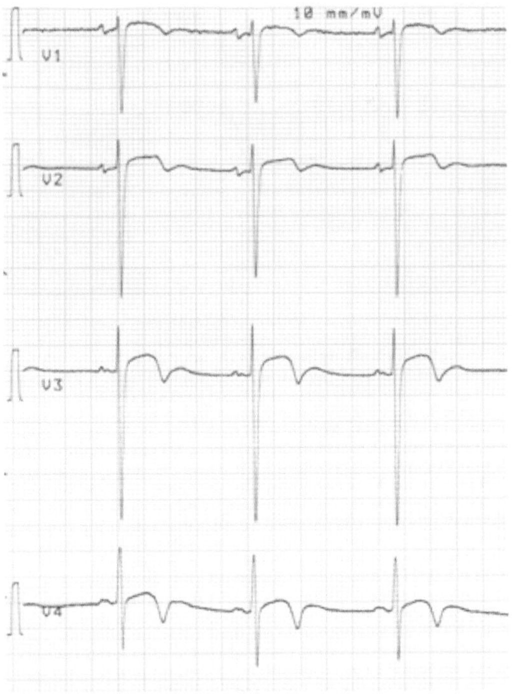

FIGURE C2.4 Resting ECG from a 19-year-old African football player showing "domed" ST elevation followed by T-wave inversion in leads V_1–V_4. Currently, this is interpreted as a normal repolarization pattern in athletes of African descent.

Committee (IOC), and the Fédération Internationale de Football Association (FIFA), uses these same methods but adds a 12-lead resting ECG.[11,24,25] In Italy, since 1982, a nationwide preparticipation screening has been mandated by law for every individual prior to getting involved in competitive sports, which has led to decades of clinical experience and outcome data.[3,4,8,26] Enhancing the sensitivity to detect cardiomyopathies, pre-excitation syndromes and ion channel disorders, among others, led to an estimated 91% increase of sensitivity to detect an underlying cardiopathy compared to the standard North American strategy.[8,27,28]

Interestingly, due to the excellent sensitivity of ECG to particularly detect hypertrophic cardiomyopathy (HCM), the most common underlying fatal cardiac disease in young athletes, as well as ARVC/D and conduction abnormalities, the addition of echocardiography to first-line screening did not result in a further increase of the sensitivity so far.[3] Effectively, the Italian/European approach has proven to decrease the annual incidence of SCD in athletes by 89%.[8]

The so-called "Seattle recommendations" are the most current and probably most accurate consensus recommendations regarding the interpretation of the 12-lead ECG in athletes.[15-18] The recommendations were developed by an international expert panel, including particularly some of the opinion leaders in the United States, where experts traditionally took up a critical position concerning the integration of the ECG in primary screening of athletes.

Once ARVC/D has been diagnosed in an athlete, restriction from most competitive sports is mandatory.[1,2] While the American expert guidelines (36th Bethesda Conference) recommend that athletes with a probable or definite diagnosis of ARVC/D should be excluded from most competitive sports, with the possible exception of those of low intensity (class IA),[2] the European guidelines recommend exclusion from any competitive sport activities.[1] Furthermore, it is essential to emphasize that prophylactic implantation of an ICD does not decrease the potential danger of the disease, particularly in association with physical exercise. Thus, the presence of an ICD in high-risk patients with cardiovascular disease should not be regarded as a protection justifying permission to participate in competitive sports that would otherwise be restricted.[1,2]

Although little evidence is available, the expert panels assert that the presence of an ICD (whether for primary or secondary prevention of SCD) should disqualify athletes from most competitive sports (with the exception of low intensity, class IA), particularly those that potentially involve body trauma.[1,2] The possibility of a sinus tachycardia triggering inappropriate shocks ultimately needs to be prevented.[1,2]

The current case report outlines another important issue: So-called "amateur" competitive athletes are mostly outside the focus regarding an adequate precompetition screening to prevent exercise-related SCD.[28,29] In a recent survey observing more than 1,000 Swiss competitive athletes who are not associated with one of the big sports associations, only a striking 9% underwent adequate cardiac screening, although their risk of SCD was relevant.[28] Particularly, female gender, younger age, and lower weekly training effort proved to be negatively associated with an adherence to screening.[28] Despite the fact that the risk for SCD in sports generally increases with age and is greater in men,[5-7,30] these subgroups of athletes need to be targeted with particular attention.

While a yearly incidence of about 0.7 to 3 SCD per 100,000 young athletes (age < 35 years) is an established estimate in literature,[5-7,30-32] newer data demonstrate a wider range. A large survey in North American marathon runners showed an unexpectedly low rate of SCD,[33] but data from North American college athletes suggested that the incidence highly depends on the kind of sports and ethnic background of an athlete.[31] For example, the risk of SCD in an African American Division I college basketball player may be as high as 1:3,000.[31]

Conclusion

In conclusion, it should once more be highlighted that ARVC/D has become a major issue in sports cardiology. However, due to continuous improvement of screening methods to prevent sudden cardiac death in competitive athletes, it should be detected in the vast majority of affected, yet asymptomatic athletes.

Abbreviations

ICD implantable cardioverter-defibrillator
RV right ventricle, right ventricular
SCD sudden cardiac death
VT ventricular tachycardia

References

1. Pelliccia A, Fagard R, Bjørnstad HH, et al. Recommendations for competitive sports participation in athletes with cardiovascular disease. *Eur Heart J*. 2005;26:1422-1445.
2. Maron BJ, Zipes DP. 36th Bethesda Conference: eligibility recommendations for competitive athletes with cardiovascular abnormalities. *J Am Coll Cardiol*. 2005;45:2-64.
3. Corrado D, Basso C, Schiavon M, Thiene G. Screening for hypertrophic cardiomyopathy in young athletes. *New Engl J Med*. 1998;339:364-369.
4. Corrado D, Thiene G, Nava A, Rossi L, Pennelli N. Sudden death in young competitive athletes: clinico-pathologic correlations in 22 cases. *Am J Med*. 1990;89:588-596.
5. Thompson PD, Funk EJ, Carleton RA, Sturner WQ. Incidence of death during jogging in Rhode Island from 1975 through 1980. *JAMA*. 1982;247:2535-2538.
6. Maron BJ. Sudden death in young athletes. *New Engl J Med*. 2003;349:1064-1075.
7. Eckart RE, Scoville SL, Campbell CL, et al. Sudden death in young adults: a 25-year review of autopsies in military recruits. *Ann Intern Med*. 2004;141:829-834.
8. Corrado D, Basso C, Pavei A, Michieli P, Schiavon M, Thiene G. Trends in sudden cardiovascular death in young competitive athletes after implementation of a preparticipation screening program. *JAMA*. 2006;296:1593-1601.
9. Fontaine G, Marcus FI, McKenna WJ, Nava A, Thiene G, Wichter T. Arrhythmogenic right ventricular dysplasia/cardiomyopathy: need for an international registry. Study Group on Arrhythmogenic Right Ventricular Dysplasia/Cardiomyopathy of the Working Groups on Myocardial and Pericardial Disease and Arrhythmias of the European Society of Cardiology and of the Scientific Council on Cardiomyopathies of the World Heart Federation. *Circulation*. 2000;101(11):E101-E106.

10. Corrado D, Schmied C, Basso C, et al. Risk of sports: do we need a pre-participation screening for competitive and leisure athletes? *Eur Heart J*. 2011;32:934-944.
11. Corrado D, Pelliccia A, Bjornstad HH, et al. Cardiovascular pre-participation screening of young competitive athletes for prevention of sudden death: proposal for a common European protocol. Consensus Statement of the Study Group of Sport Cardiology of the Working Group of Cardiac Rehabilitation and Exercise Physiology and the Working Group of Myocardial and Pericardial Diseases of the European Society of Cardiology. *Eur Heart J*. 2005;26:516-524.
12. Maron BJ, Thompson PD, Ackerman MJ, et al. Recommendations and considerations related to preparticipation screening for cardiovascular abnormalities in competitive athletes: 2007 update: a scientific statement from the American Heart Association Council on Nutrition, Physical Activity, and Metabolism: endorsed by the American College of Cardiology Foundation. *Circulation*. 2007;115:1643-1655. http://circ.ahajournals.org/content/115/12/1643.full.pdf
13. Corrado D, Pelliccia A, Heidbuchel H, et al. Section of Sports Cardiology, European Association of Cardiovascular Prevention and Rehabilitation. Recommendations for interpretation of 12-lead electrocardiogram in the athlete. *Eur Heart J*. 2010;31(2):243-259.
14. Uberoi A, Stein R, Perez MV, et al. Interpretation of the electrocardiogram of young athletes. *Circulation*. 2011;124(6):746-757.
15. Drezner JA, Ackerman MJ, Anderson J, et al. Electrocardiographic interpretation in athletes: the "Seattle criteria." *Br J Sports Med*. 2013;47(3):122-124.
16. Drezner JA, Fischbach P, Froelicher V, et al. Normal electrocardiographic findings: recognising physiological adaptations in athletes. *Br J Sports Med*. 2013;47(3):125-136.
17. Drezner JA, Ackerman MJ, Cannon BC, et al. Abnormal electrocardiographic findings in athletes: recognising changes suggestive of primary electrical disease. *Br J Sports Med*. 2013;47(3):153-167.
18. Drezner JA, Ashley E, Baggish AL, et al. Abnormal electrocardiographic findings in athletes: recognising changes suggestive of cardiomyopathy. *Br J Sports Med*. 2013;47(3): 137-152.
19. Marcus FI, McKenna WJ, Sherrill D, et al. Diagnosis of arrhythmogenic right ventricular cardiomyopathy/dysplasia (ARVC/D). *Circulation*. 2010;121(13):1533-1541.
20. Jain R, Dalal D, Daly A, et al. electrocardiographic features of arrhythmogenic right ventricular dysplasia. *Circulation*. 2009; 120(6):477.
21. Schmied C, Zerguini Y, Junge A, et al. Cardiac findings in the precompetition medical assessment of football players participating in the 2009 African Under-17 Championships in Algeria. *Br J Sports Med*. 2009;43(9):716-721.
22. Papadakis M, Carre F, Kervio G, et al. The prevalence, distribution and clinical outcomes of electrocardiographic repolarisation patterns in male athletes of African/Afro-Caribbean origin. *Eur Heart J*. 2011;32:2304-2313.
23. Di Paolo FM, Schmied C, Zerguini AY, et al. The athlete's heart in adolescent Africans: electrocardiographic and echocardiographic study. *J Am Coll Cardiol*. 2012;59(11):1029-1036.
24. Dvorak J, Grimm K, Schmied C, Junge A. Development and implementation of a standardized precompetition medical assessment of international elite football players. *Clin J Sport Med*. 2009;19(4):316-321.
25. Bille K, Figueiras D, Schamasch P, et al. Sudden cardiac death in athletes: the Lausanne Recommendations. *Eur J Cardiovasc Prev Rehabil*. 2006;13(6):859-875.
26. Corrado D, Basso C, Rizzoli G, Schiavon M, Thiene G. Does sports activity enhance the risk of sudden death in adolescents and young adults? *J Am Coll Cardiol*. 2003;42: 1959-1963.
27. Pelliccia A, Di Paolo FM, Corrado D, et al. Evidence for efficacy of the Italian national pre-participation screening programme for identification of hypertrophic cardiomyopathy in competitive athletes. *Eur Heart J*. 2006;27:2196-2200.

28. Schmied C, Notz S, Cribari M, et al. Cardiac pre-competition screening in Swiss athletes. *Swiss Med Wkly*. 2012;142:w13575.
29. Schwotzer R, Kistler W, Keller DI, et al. Optimizing cardiac pre-competition screening in competitive amateur athletes. *Swiss Med Wkly*. 2013 May 7;143:w13785.
30. Maron BJ, Doerer JJ, Haas TS, Tierney DM, Mueller FO. Sudden deaths in young competitive athletes: analysis of 1866 deaths in the United States, 1980-2006. *Circulation*. 2009;119:1085-1092.
31. Harmon KG, Asif IM, Klossner D, Drezner JA. Incidence of sudden cardiac death in national collegiate athletic association athletes. *Circulation*. 2011;123(15):1594-1600.
32. Meyer L, Stubbs B, Fahrenbruch C, et al. Incidence, causes, and survival trends from cardiovascular-related sudden cardiac arrest in children and young adults 0 to 35 years of age: a 30-year review. *Circulation*. 2012;126(11):1363-1372.
33. Kim JH, Malhotra R, Chiampas G, et al. Race Associated Cardiac Arrest Event Registry (RACER) study group. *N Engl J Med*. 2012;366(2):130-140.

Impressions from the First Zurich ARVC/D Symposium

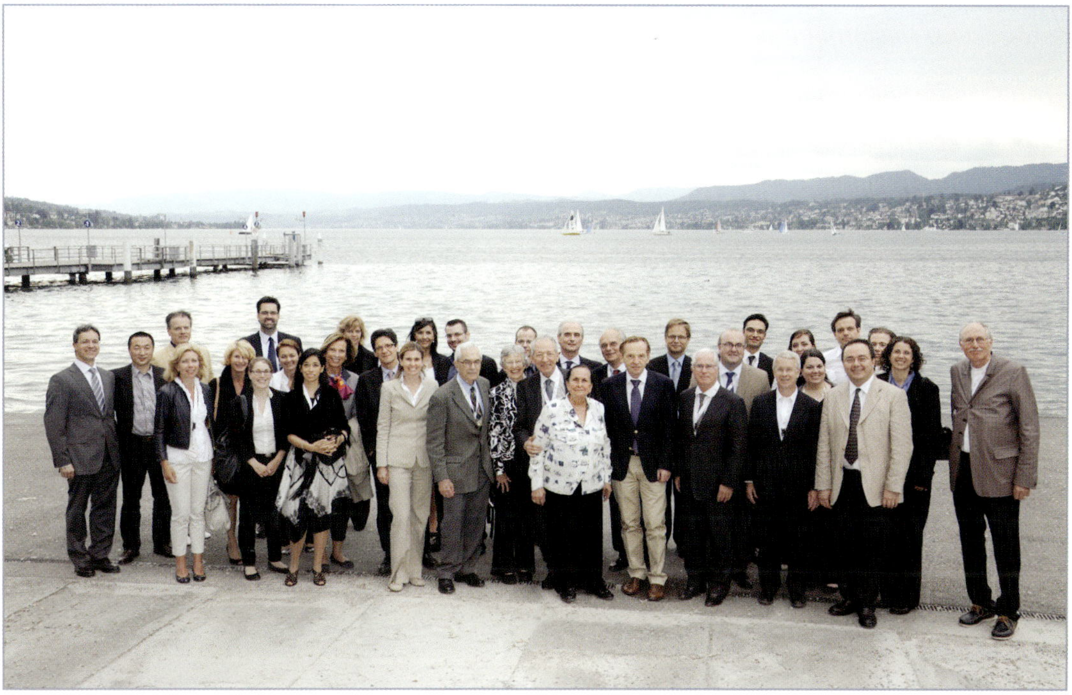

IMPRESSIONS FROM THE FIRST ZURICH ARVC/D SYMPOSIUM, LAKE ZURICH, MAY 2012.

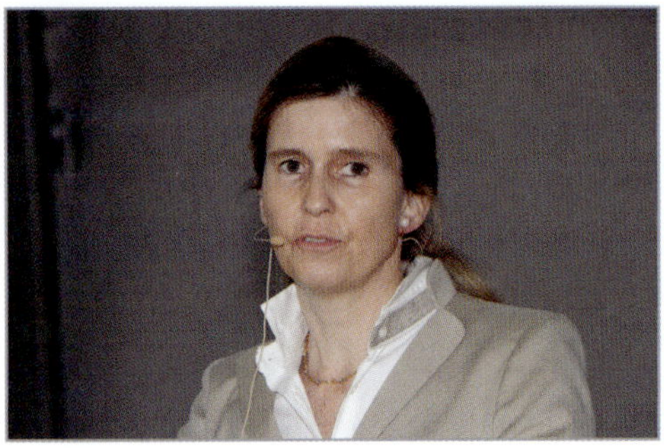

CORINNA BRUNCKHORST

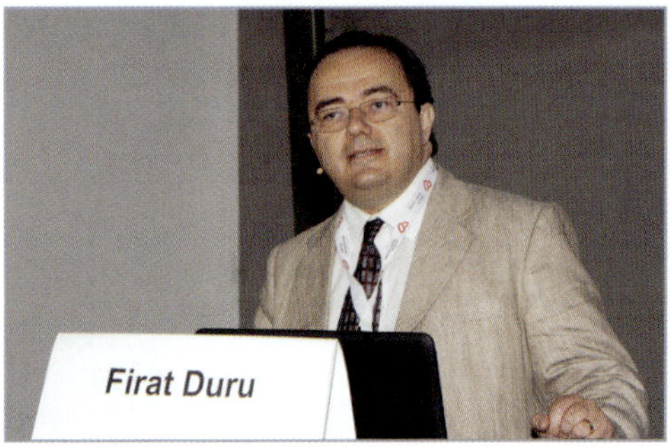

FIRAT DURU

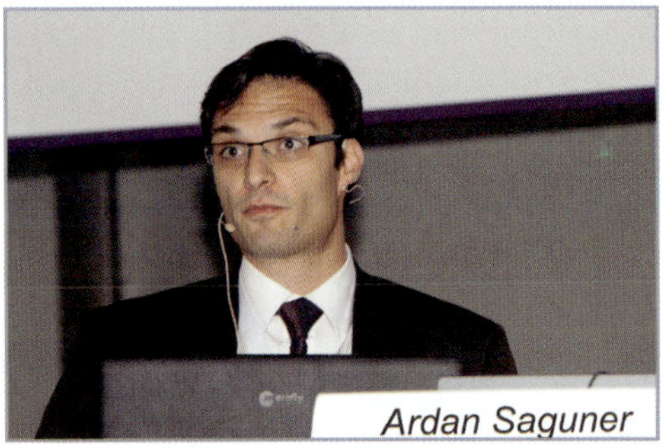

ARDAN M. SAGUNER

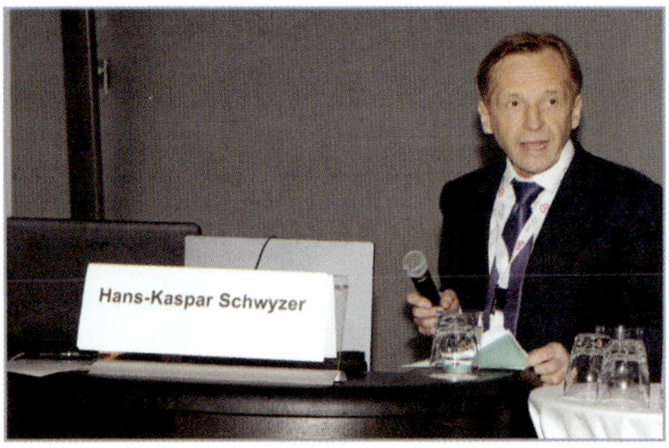

HANS-KASPAR SCHWYZER, GEORG AND BERTHA SCHWYZER-WINIKER FOUNDATION

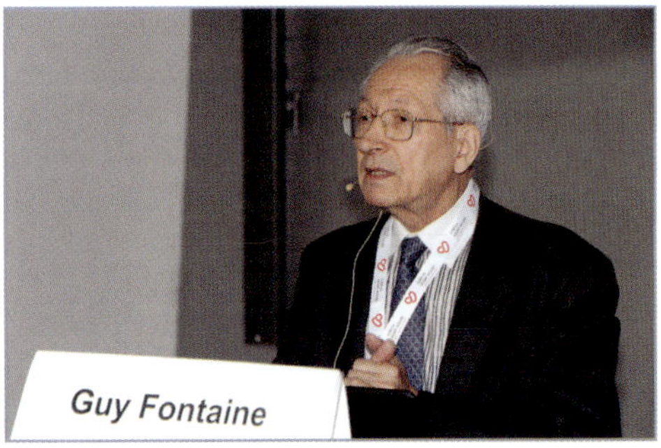

GUY H. FONTAINE

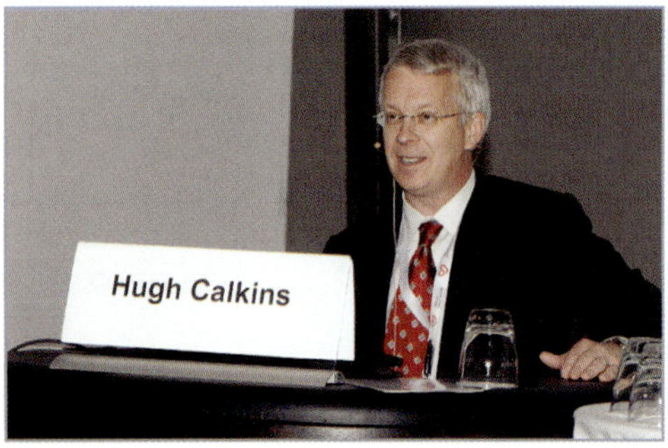

HUGH CALKINS

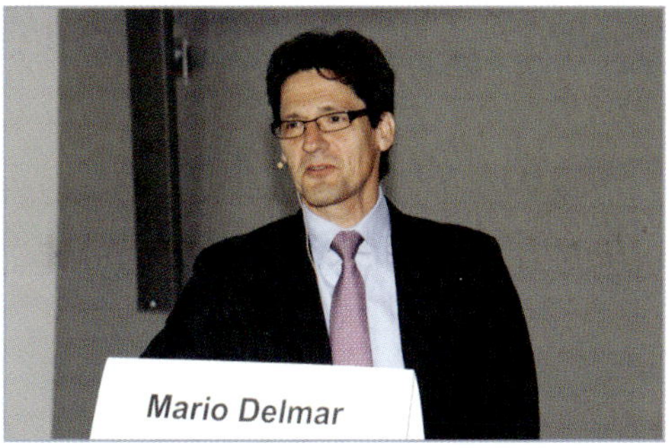

MARIO DELMAR

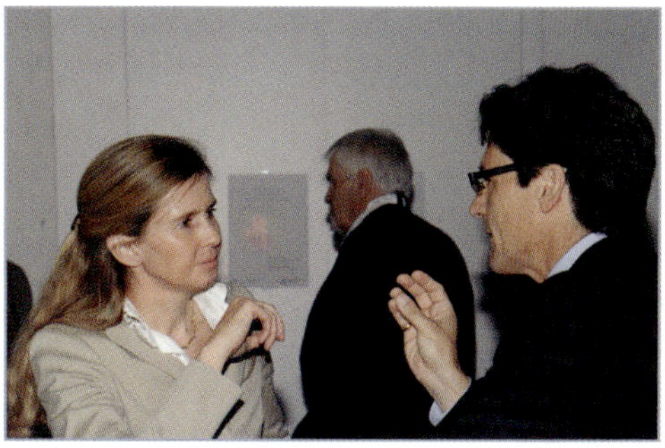

CORINNA BRUNCKHORST (left) and MARIO DELMAR (right)

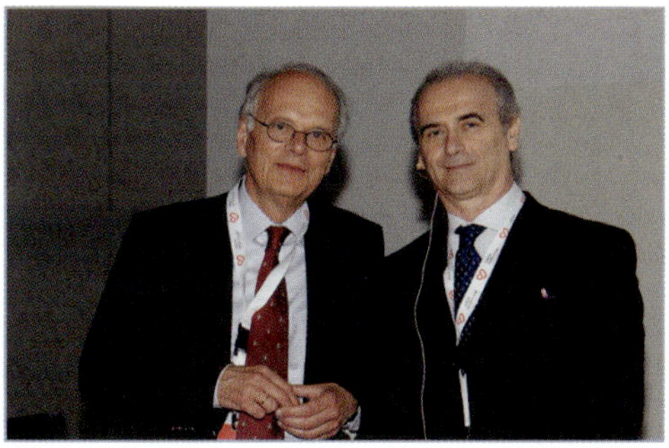

RICHARD HAUER (left) and DOMENICO CORRADO (right)

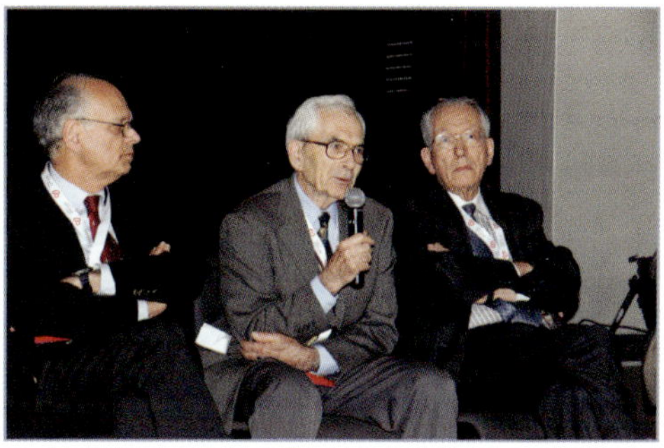

RICHARD HAUER (left), FRANK I. MARCUS (center), and GUY H. FONTAINE (right)

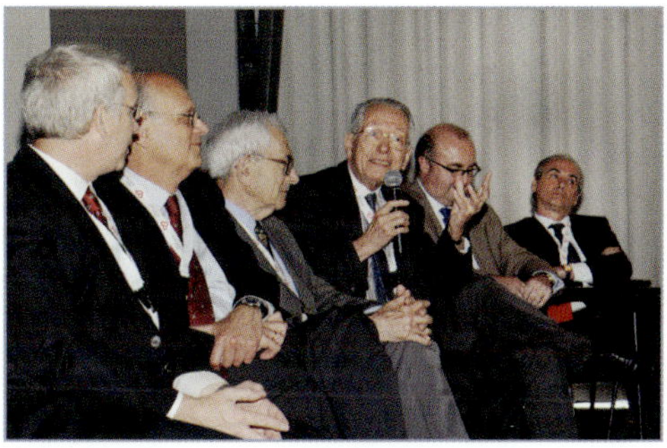

(From left) HUGH CALKINS, RICHARD HAUER, FRANK I. MARCUS, GUY H. FONTAINE, THOMAS WICHTER, and DOMENICO CORRADO

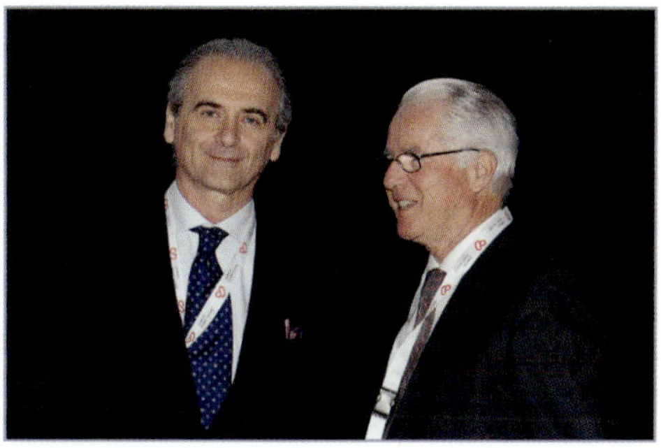

DOMENICO CORRADO (left) and LUKAS KAPPENBERGER (right)

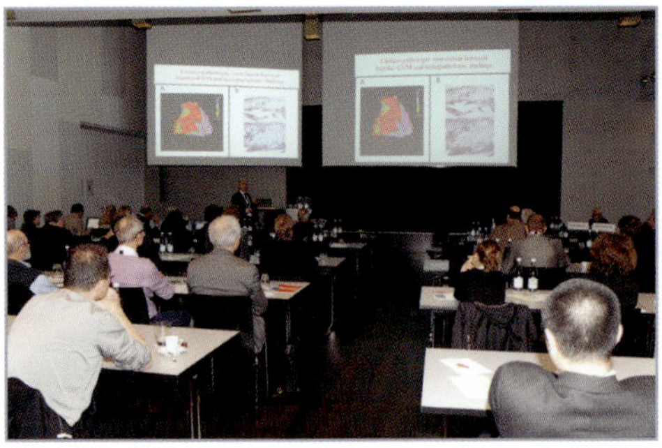

DOMENICO CORRADO SPEAKING IN FRONT OF THE AUDIENCE

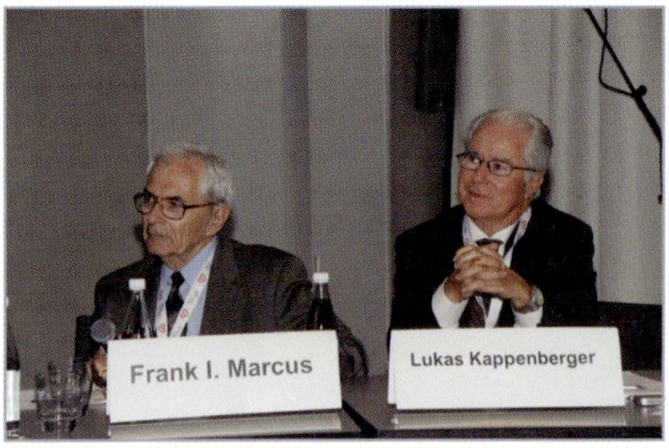

FRANK I. MARCUS (left) and LUKAS KAPPENBERGER (right)

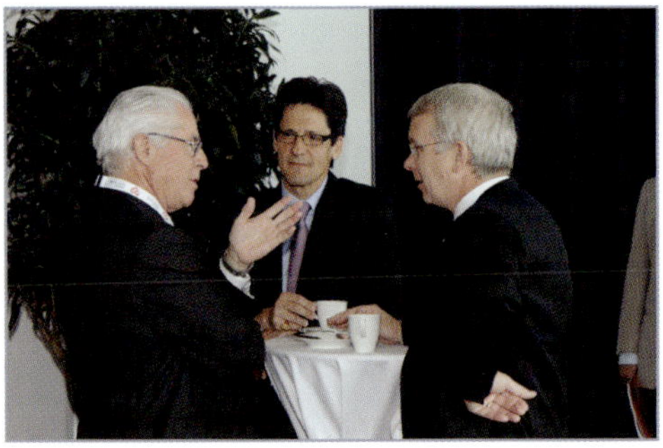

LUKAS KAPPENBERGER (left), MARIO DELMAR (center), and HUGH CALKINS (right)

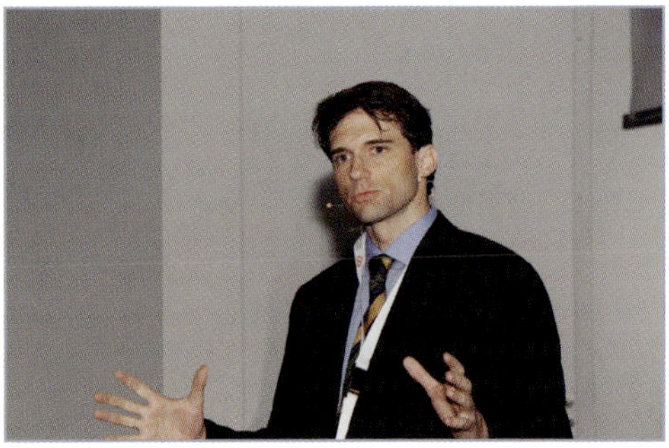

CHRISTIAN M. SCHMIED

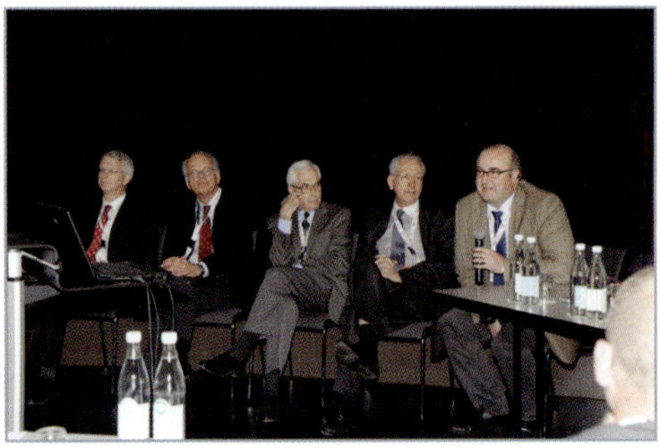

From left to right: HUGH CALKINS, RICHARD HAUER, FRANK I. MARCUS, GUY H. FONTAINE, and THOMAS WICHTER

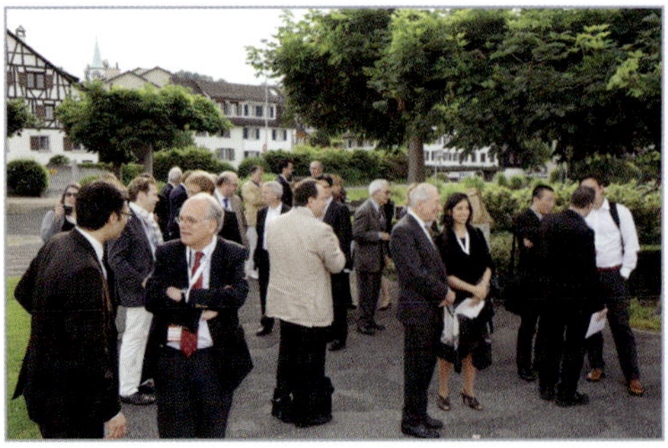

GROUP PHOTO IN RÜSCHLIKON, WHERE THE SYMPOSIUM TOOK PLACE

Index

D

E

J

L

M

N

O

P

Q

R

S

T